Cancer: Don't Drop the Mic!

Lessons Learned, Opportunities Opened,
and Purposes Pursued
on the Treatment Trail

William and Cynthia Bartlett

Dove Christian Publishers
Bladensburg, MD

Dove Christian Publishers
P.O. Box 611
Bladensburg, MD 20710-0611
www.dovechristianpublishers.com

Library of Congress Control Number: 2016956963

ISBN: 978-0-9975898-3-2

Printed in the United States of America

Cover and Interior Photography by William Bartlett

Additional photography (c) Mipam | Dreamstime.com

Cancer: Don't Drop the Mic!

Table of Contents

Foreword

Part One—Background

Part Two— Lessons Learned, Opportunities Opened, Purposes Pursued

Foreword

Cancer comes with lessons, opportunities, purposes—and responsibilities.

Cancer teaches lessons—fast. There is an immediate seriousness to life when the diagnosis of cancer is received. Maturity and perspective that often take decades seem to dawn overnight in cancer patients.

Cancer opens opportunities. Family, friends, coworkers, and even strangers stop, pause, and listen to newly diagnosed cancer patients. Well, if you're the patient, what are you going to say?

Cancer pings a patient for purpose in his or her life. Without purpose in life, cancer treatment—life itself—is pointless, aimless, and an empty waste of time. But, with purpose in life, even cancer and its treatment become opportunities to punctuate life with impact, meaning, and significance.

Cancer also comes with a mantle of responsibility. Cancer is an attention-getter, both for the patient and for those within the patient's sphere of influence. Part of the reason why people around the patient are often silent in the presence of the patient with cancer is that they are listening. They want to hear words of wisdom, insights gained, and admonitions that compellingly come from someone who speaks from the perspective of facing eternity. So, dear fellow-patient, DON'T DROP THE MIC! Say something! And, not just something. Speak words worthy of the perspective that cancer gives. Talk of your faith in the Lord. Talk about new insights, priorities, challenges, and opportunities that have flooded like a torrent into your life. Make the most of the opportunity you have. Be a faithful steward of the opportunities (yes, opportunities) that have come, and will come, because of cancer. In some odd and ironic way, cancer can make a person more alive than he or she was before diagnosis. Charge into this new journey with the excitement of a pioneer—knowing that our Lord "goes before us and is with us" and that Jesus is the first "Pioneer ... Who for the joy that was set before Him [referring to our salvation and healing] endured the cross" (Hebrews 12:2). With that assurance, come what may, all is OK!

Acts 20:24 has become my new theme life-verse since diagnosis: "I consider my life worth nothing to me; my only aim is to finish the race and complete the task the Lord Jesus has given me—the task of testifying to the good news of God's grace."

Fellow-patient or caregiver, the world is listening for us to speak. DON'T DROP THE MIC!

This book has four parts:

1. Part One sets the context and stage for Part Two. The background of my journey with cancer, from diagnosis to current treatment, is summarized, emphasizing and detailing how this journey has taught me lessons, opened opportunities, and thrust a microphone into my hands. My family, friends, and even unexpected spheres of observers are watching and listening as I engage, grow from, and embrace the lessons, opportunities, and purposes that this journey brings. Everyone, at some time, will face a journey like this. How can my journey prepare them for theirs?

2. Part Two lists "Lessons Learned, Opportunities Opened, and Purposed Pursued on the Treatment Trail." Each lesson, opportunity, or purpose shared in this section, in the text boxes, has been an entry in a journey that I started at diagnosis in August 2013, and in which I continue to make entries. Following the text box, I have added brief reflections or expansions on each entry. Several entries in my journal have Internet links to supporting or resulting documents. The e-Book version contains live links to many of these references.

3. Part Three contains reflections from a caregiver—Cindy, my wife, who tenderly, sacrificially, patiently, and always lovingly supported me, sat next to me (fully exposed to high dose chemotherapy while the nurses, in full protective

gowning, administered drugs), faithfully drove to and from the hospital (sometimes taking five hours a day), and carried the full weight of a household during times of my weakness.

4. Part Four contains two QR codes to access my ongoing list of "Lessons Learned, Opportunities Opened, and Purposes Pursued" and to open an ongoing "Don't Drop the Mic!" blog for cancer patients, caregivers, and loved ones for the purpose of keeping our dialog with, and support of, each other alive!

Special thanks to my wife, Cindy, to my children and grandchildren, and to close friends who have been a huge part of that "cloud of witnesses" (Hebrews 12:1) surrounding me with love, TLC, compassion, company, prayers, and purpose for living boldly and in the eternal and strong presence and promises of our Lord Jesus Christ. Special thanks also to Dove Christian Publishers (www.dovechristianpublishers.com) for their professional and faithful partnership in bringing my manuscript to publication. They have demonstrated a consistent pursuit of their mission, which is "to glorify Jesus Christ while entertaining, edifying, encouraging and exhorting the Church."

If you are reading this book, chances are pretty good that you are a cancer patient, or you know and love a cancer patient. In either case, this journey has given you and will give you lessons to be learned, opportunities to be opened, and purposes to be pursued—all of which become your responsibility to share!

It is my prayer that one message becomes clear to you through this book:

DON'T DROP THE MIC! The world is listening!

Part One—Background

It was August 2013, when the Lord turned my world upside down and handed me a microphone—in the form of a call from my doctor while I was at work. My doctor said, "You've got cancer." The situation spoke another frightening and yet compelling message to me, "Along with cancer, you've also got a microphone!"

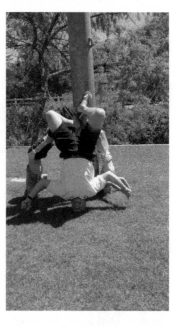

"Don't Drop the Mic!"

The phrase, "Drop the mic," at least in urban usage, usually means that such a compelling statement is made that no further comment is warranted. In the matter of cancer treatment, there can never be a "Drop the Mic" moment. Constant, ongoing conversation is needed, appreciated, and part of the treatment process.

This book is a compilation of "Lessons Learned, Opportunities Opened, and Purposes Pursued" through my experience and journey with cancer since my diagnosis in August 2013. The purposes of sharing these learnings are to comfort and help fellow-travelers on the cancer treatment trail, to keep the pump primed so my cancer-afflicted colleagues will keep sharing their experiences and learnings, and to encourage all of us to heed the admonition, "Don't Drop the Mic"—to the praise and glory of our Lord Jesus Christ.

At the time of my diagnosis in August 2013, I had been a pastor for 38 years. I was used to having captive audiences on Sunday mornings. But, after my diagnosis, I sensed that people were listening more closely than ever before.

Why were people listening so attentively after my cancer diagnosis, and why are people still listening? The Celtic Christians from Ireland used to speak of "thin places." The phrase "thin places" referred to both times and places when and where there seemed to be a "thinning" of the separation between mortal life and eternal life. "Thin places," therefore, are holy places. People listen when they sense a "thin place" because all people are aware of their own mortality.

We Are All in the Same Mortal Line.

We all know, but hate to think about the fact, that we all—ALL!—are in the same mortal line. We often suppress that awareness:

- In youth and young adulthood, because the threat or reality of death seems an eternity away;
- In middle age, because we are too busy just surviving the busyness we let co-opt our lives;
- And in old age because of fear or denial of what happens after death.

Since my diagnosis in August 2013, I have kept track, on my prayer list, of people I have known who have died. I thought, back in August 2013, that I was at the front of the "mortality" line among everyone I knew. Yet, since that date, I have known eight people who have died. And, here's the shocker: I'm still here, and four of those eight have been under 25 years of age. None of us knows where we are in that "mortality line"; but one thing is certain—we are all in that line!

Deep within every person is that nagging realization which King David and his son, the wisest man in the world, Solomon, knew well:

- "There is but a step between me and death" (1 Sam. 20:3).
- "He has also set eternity in the human heart" (Eccl. 3:11).

There is no denying it, repressing it, running from it, or outsmarting it. Death and eternity are realities which confront us all and which compel us to face our own mortality.

Try as we may to hide death and eternity behind a thick curtain, cancer and other life-threatening illnesses draw the curtain open on these topics and often reveal either a dropped mic pretending that there is nothing to say, or a stage, a mic, and a podium with a listening and attentive audience, anxious to hear what lessons and experiences we have to speak about life, death, and eternity. When this happens in your life, "Don't Drop the Mic!"

My Background and Treatment Trail

- August 2013: Diagnosed with Hodgkin's Lymphoma.
- September 2013: Stepped away from my ministry as founding executive director at Crean Lutheran High School to focus on treatment.
- September 2013 - February 2014: ABVD chemotherapy treatments at UCLA, with an optimistic perspective due to a 90% cure rate with this treatment protocol.
- August 2014: Diagnosed with recurrent Hodgkin's Lymphoma (10% of those treated with ABVD chemotherapy for Hodgkin's Lymphoma have a recurrence). Treatment: stem cell transplant.
  - August-October, 2014: RICE & BEAM chemotherapy prior to stem cell transplant at UCLA.
  - October 27, 2014: Stem cell transplant at UCLA (50% of stem cell patients are cured; 50% have a recurrence within one year).
- May 22, 2015: PET/CT scan showed that the Hodgkin's Lymphoma returned. Treatment: a clinical trial using Bristol-Myers Squibb's immunotherapy drug, Opdivo.

- June 5, 2015: Screening tests for enrollment in UCLA clinical trial using a new drug called Opdivo.
- June 23, 2015—current (as of the writing of this book): Started Clinical Trial using a new drug, Opdivo, which I receive every two weeks. I am one among approximately 300 patients worldwide, in about a dozen sites, participating in this 2nd phase, FDA registrational trial, praying that this new immunotherapy will become a new, effective, patient-friendly, and durable front-line treatment for many types of cancer in place of the current and harsher front line treatments of surgery, chemotherapy, and radiation.

Lessons Learned, Opportunities Opened, and Purposes Pursued

Upon diagnosis, back in 2013, I knew that I was in for a journey. So, I began a journal which evolved into the "Lessons Learned, Opportunities Opened, and Purposes Pursued on the Treatment Trail" listed in this book. Lessons are still being learned, opportunities are still being opened, and new purposes continually point me in new directions. These continuing lessons, opportunities, and purposes are then added to my journal. This book, therefore, is a snapshot of this living journey from August 2013 until the time of completion of this manuscript. Over these 36 months, I have made approximately 90 entries in this journal— about one entry every week and a half. I expect this pattern to continue as the Lord is faithful to teach me and, I pray, use me to "make the most of every opportunity" (Col. 4:5)—even this opportunity—to lean on Him, to proclaim Jesus' saving grace, and to encourage and comfort others in their sufferings and treatment all the while our Lord provides for and comforts me.

The purposes of this book are:

- To stimulate discussion about cancer treatment.
- To encourage those on the treatment trail and to assure them of the sufficiency of Jesus for the journey.
- To give purpose to cancer patients as they share their lessons learned with others and respond with impact to opportunities opened.
- And to boldly speak an admonition to everyone, "DON'T DROP THE MIC!"

In Part Two of this book, I share the many Lessons Learned, Opportunities Opened, and Purposes Pursued that have impacted my life, that have given meaning and purpose to my life even during this journey, and that have, by God's grace, been a positive encouragement to others, either patients or loved ones, on the treatment trail! In my online journal, several of the Lessons Learned, Opportunities Opened, and Purposes Pursued contain links to other resources or documents related to each Lesson, Opportunity, or Purpose. Also, as stated in the Foreword, at the end of this book are QR codes which link to my actual and growing Journal and to a "Don't Drop the Mic!" blog. I invite readers to access these documents to read ongoing and additional Lessons, Opportunities, and Purposes, and to join a blog in which they too can share with others their Lessons Learned, Opportunities Opened, and Purposes Pursued.

Ephesians 6:19 well communicates my prayer for this book and for my life's passion on this journey:

> "Pray also for me, that whenever I speak [or write!],
> words may be given me so that I will fearlessly make
> known the mystery of the Gospel...."

Please join me in "making known" the Lessons we are learning and then sharing these Lessons through the Opportunities and Purposes that are opened as together we respond to the admonition, **"DON'T DROP THE MIC!"**

Part Two— Lessons Learned, Opportunities Opened, Purposes Pursued

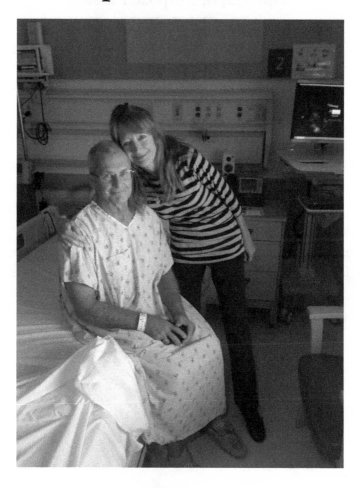

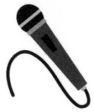

1 Jesus is the Treasure

Lesson Learned, Opportunity Opened, or Purpose Pursued:

Jesus is the Treasure, not the Bearer of the Treasure. Jesus is Greater than Health, Healing, or Any Earthly Blessing.

This journey has unmasked a common misconception held by many Christians—including me—prior to cancer. So often my prayers have been very selfish: "Lord, please forgive ME, please heal ME, please open this door for ME," and on and on.

Even Lazarus, after his sisters' pleas for him and our Lord's gracious response of restoring him to life, died a physical death sometime later. The real gift, the greatest gift, the only gift, blessing, and reality that really matters is Jesus.

Indeed, Jesus is far more than the Giver, the Bearer, the Author of earthly blessings. JESUS is the Treasure. With Jesus will come forgiveness, life, and eternal salvation. That is ... He is! ... the greatest treasure.

Have Jesus and you have all that really matters.

2 Jesus is Sufficient

Lesson Learned, Opportunity Opened, or Purpose Pursued:

Jesus is Sufficient, Even More than Sufficient, for Anything We Face in Life.

Oh, it seems close sometimes. The discomfort of chemotherapy, or the multiple sticks to start an IV, or the hearing of not as good news as you had hoped after a PET-CT scan can all leave you occasionally wondering, "Are You really sufficient?"

And, yes Jesus is. Somehow, He brings strength through my wife, or an email or a card from a friend, or simply through His Holy Word or powerful Spirit. And, I reach shore again, the storm stills, and peace returns.

The Lord said, "My grace is sufficient" (2 Corinthians 12:9).

After feeding the 5,000, Jesus made sure His disciples knew there were twelve baskets of leftovers. More than sufficient.

After promising that we will never be tested beyond what we can bear, our Lord promises that if it does get too hot in the furnace, He will provide a way out. That's a more than sufficient Savior.

Our Lord Jesus sees that we may not always get or have or experience or be what we want, but always what we need—even more than sufficient.

Our world tempts us to think that more is always better; Jesus teaches us that He—and He alone—is sufficient.

3 The Lord said, "Go...."

Lesson Learned, Opportunity Opened, or Purpose Pursued:

> The Lord Said, "Go ... to the Place I will Show You,"
> "I am With You Always."

"Go from your country, your people and your father's household to the place I will show you" (Gen. 12:1).

"Go and make disciples of all nations, baptizing them in the name of the Father and of the Son and of the Holy Spirit, and teaching them to obey everything I have commanded you. And surely I am with you always, to the very end of the age" (Matthew 28:19-20).

Our Lord has a habit of Calling and Sending. He calls us to come to Him. He then tells us to go places we often had not wished to go! But, in going where He sends us, there is the peace, joy, and strength of knowing that Jesus "goes with us."

In August 2013, our Lord Called me from a busy and exciting life of a Christian high school administrator and pastor to "go" to a place I had no desire going—to a world of cancer, chemotherapy, and ongoing challenges.

May I journey to every place our Lord sends me in the peace of the promise of Deuteronomy 31:8,

> "The Lord Himself goes before you and will be with you; He will never leave you nor forsake you. Do not be afraid; do not be discouraged."

4 Even this!

Lesson Learned, Opportunity Opened, or Purpose Pursued:

> "I Can do All Things Through Him Who Strengthens Me." Even this!

The above passage is from Philippians 4:13. I grew up with a limited, inaccurate, and (confession coming!) very selfish understanding of this verse. For some reason (probably my own self-centeredness), I had always understood this verse to mean that I (emphasis on me!) could do anything I wanted because the Lord would give me strength to do it.

I was wrong on several counts. First, the Lord doesn't want me to do some things that I want to do. Second, the Lord is not interested in making me into a Superman with superhuman strength or qualities. And, third, the Lord knows that my sinful, human, weak nature is in desperate need for His daily (hourly! Minute by minute!) strength.

The Lord showed me that life serves up many dishes that are not to our liking or taste. The Lord promises that "in this world you will have trouble" (John 16:33). The Lord has demonstrated and revealed to me that "through Him" I can even endure cancer, chemotherapy, a stem cell transplant, and disappointment after disappointment, because He strengthens me. It is His strength, not mine, that enables me to do—even this cancer treatment.

Blaise Pascal, the great mathematician and scientist, after coming to faith, wrote about the integration of the Lord's presence and power with his own scientific pursuits and achievements in a short prayer that we all would do well to remember and pray daily:

> "Lord, help me to do great and difficult things as though they were little and simple, since I do them with Your

power; and little things as though they were great and important, since I do them in Your name." (paraphrase)

Here is a Bible verse that strengthens me regularly:

"To this end I labor with all His energy which works so powerfully within me" (Col. 1:29).

5 Be Pre-prayered!

Lesson Learned, Opportunity
Opened, or Purpose Pursued:

> Daily Prayer is a Priority and is Powerful.

This journey has changed, enhanced, and compelled my prayer life. I will paste the first several petitions (and priorities) of my daily prayer list below. It is interesting to me that the highest priorities in my prayer life do not change. These first petitions are not affected by the lesser issues (i.e., asking for help for a specific matter, asking for guidance in a decision, and even asking for healing from cancer) that occupy the next specific petitions section of my prayer list.

Here are the first petitions—and priorities—for my daily prayers:

- Thanks and praise to You for:
    - Salvation purchased through Christ Who died in payment for my and all people's sins, and then rose from the dead, offering me and all people eternal life;
    - The gift of the Bible, Your self-disclosure and revelation to us;
    - The peace and presence of the Holy Spirit;
    - Your all-sufficiency in all circumstances; and
    - The certainty of eternal life with Christ and all the saints.
- Thank You for Cindy—for her care, her support, her love, and our marriage.
- Please grant blessings, grace, forgiveness, regeneration in You, and strength for me to be a faithful disciple and a winsome witness to You during this time.

- Thank You for a faithful and loving family.

Following these weightier petitions, I then proceed to pray some specific petitions:

- To be healed through this treatment, to have a significant holy, happy, healthy, and Kingdom-furthering next season, with Cindy, serving and proclaiming You.
- That, by Your agency, successful treatment through Opdivo will occur allowing Cindy and me to serve You as You enable us; and, if not, that some other effective treatment will be available; and, if not, that even still I may be a winsome witness to You. But yet, I pray for a cure because You are powerful, able, loving, and You invite us to come to You with specific requests in prayer—and because You, if it be within Your Will, can make Opdivo, by itself or in combination, be an effective first-line treatment for many.
- To have and reflect the joy of the Lord.
- Pray through the day's events.

Thank You, Jesus, that You invite us to pray, that You promise to hear our prayers, and that You promise to answer our prayers. Amen.

6 Opportunity!

Lesson Learned, Opportunity Opened, or Purpose Pursued:

> Don't Waste the Opportunity!

Don't waste the opportunity—even responsibility!—and don't drop the microphone in using, learning from, and sharing from, this experience for deepening our relationships with Christ, and for taking advantage of the fact that others are listening, watching, noticing, and potentially ready to be affected by our stewardship of this journey.

Share the lessons learned. Boldly enter the opportunities opened. Let renewed purpose be pursued as we strive to find meaning and significance even in this journey!

"Thanks be to God, Who always leads us as captives in Christ's triumphal procession and uses us to spread the aroma of the knowledge of Him everywhere" (2 Cor. 2:14).

Dear Lord, may I be a fragrant witness to You to others.

7 The Mortality Line

Lesson Learned, Opportunity Opened, or Purpose Pursued:

Everyone (EVERYONE!) is in the Same Mortal Line!

Who knows who will die next? It could be you. It could be me. It could be a family member or a friend. We never really know our place in that line of human mortality.

Some of us—especially those of us in this journey of cancer treatment—think that we may be near the front of this line. Some others, especially those in their 20s, 30s, and 40s, think they are far back in the line.

We who are at, or even appear to be at, the front of the line have responsibilities and opportunities for those following. Our job—and privilege—is to encourage them to live in the light of eternity even now. That means to take the Lord Jesus seriously, even now.

As of this date, eight people, in my circle, who were healthy when I was diagnosed in August 2013, have died. FOUR of them were under twenty-five years of age!

Indeed, we never know where we are in this line of human mortality. No one does! Therefore, let us live in light of eternity every day—and invite others to do the same!

8 Mission Unchanged!

Lesson Learned, Opportunity Opened, or Purpose Pursued:

> My Personal Mission Statement—Unchanged!

Here is an interesting learning and observation that recently came to me:

> My Personal Mission Statement (purpose) has not changed through all of this.

Approximately twenty-five years ago, I wrote and adopted a Personal Mission Statement. The act was motivated by a retreat in which I was participating. During the retreat, we all were invited to write a Mission Statement for the church we were serving. We were all pastors of local congregations. During the exercise of writing a mission statement for our church, it struck me (like a ton of bricks!) that if a church had a Mission Statement, and if all major companies (from Coca-Cola to Apple) had Mission Statements, shouldn't my life also have a purpose—or mission statement?

That very moment, I began to craft my Mission Statement:

- Created by God, lost through sin, redeemed by Christ, and regenerated and daily refined by the Holy Spirit, I daily strive to glorify the Lord, to be a faithful steward of all that God has entrusted to my care, and to winsomely share Jesus Christ with as many people as possible.

At the beginning of my cancer diagnosis, I added this verse as an addendum to my Mission Statement:

- "I consider my life worth nothing to me, if only I may finish the race and complete the task the Lord Jesus has given me —the task of testifying to the Gospel of God's grace" (Acts 20:24).

This journey of cancer and its treatment have not lessened, changed, or hindered my Mission. In many ways, this journey has facilitated it!

9 So What? So That!

Lesson Learned, Opportunity Opened, or Purpose Pursued:

> We are Comforted SO THAT We Can Comfort Others!

How wrong, inconsiderate, selfish, and short-sighted would I be if I did not pass on to others what I have.

No, I'm of course not talking about the cancer; I'm talking about the God-given compassion and comfort that our Lord is providing in more-than-sufficient measure.

One reason our Lord has poured out this compassion and comfort is simply His amazing grace.

Another reason our Lord has poured out this compassion and comfort is "so that" (note the purpose, the obligation, the conscription!) I will share these blessings with others.

> "Praise be to the God and Father of our Lord Jesus Christ, the Father of compassion and the God of all comfort, Who comforts us in all our troubles, <u>so that</u> we can comfort those in any trouble with the comfort we ourselves receive from God. For just as we share abundantly in the sufferings of Christ, so also our comfort abounds through Christ" (2 Cor. 1:3-5).

10 Count Your Blessings!

Lesson Learned, Opportunity
Opened, or Purpose Pursued:

Count Blessings & Building Blocks—Daily!

During this cancer journey, my wife and I made a practice of daily recounting three blessings. It is like a game, except it is serious. We each alternate listing one blessing at a time until each of us lists three blessings.

- Blessings are gifts from our Lord.
- Examples: Christ's presence and purpose in my life, company of loved ones, beauty in creation (sunset, beaches, foliage, conversations), cards or phone calls received, good medical care, caregivers, God's precious Word, the gift of Christian music, etc.

On a personal level, I also have made an effort to lay at least three Building Blocks each day.

- Building Blocks are our constructive deeds and participation in the coming Kingdom of Christ.
- Examples: care-calls to others in need (ill, hurting, etc.), cards or emails or texts of encouragement, visits or small gifts or expressions of thanks and love, service and outreach projects meeting physical or spiritual needs, etc.

Blessings and Building Blocks enhance and beautify any life!

11 My Concerns Versus the Lord's Ultimate Concern

Lesson Learned, Opportunity Opened, or Purpose Pursued:

> I May Be Concerned about How Things Turn Out. Jesus is More Concerned about How I Turn Out. -Philip Yancey, <u>The Question that Never Goes Away</u>, (paraphrase)

When we are in any need—a predicament at work, a relationship issue with a loved one, or a medical condition in which we now find ourselves—we are often obsessed with "how things turn out."

When I read the above quote in Philip Yancey's book, <u>The Question that Never Goes Away</u>, I was indicted. What a short-sighted perspective I was holding.

Shouldn't I, instead, be concerned about how I will be refined, chastened, purified, sanctified, and made better through this journey as I relied more and more deeply on the Lord?

I'm not saying that the Lord set me on this path to "teach me a lesson." Rather, believing in the sovereignty, power, and goodness of our Lord, I am saying that Jesus can use this journey for good—for my good, and for the good of others around me.

> "We know that for those who love God all things work together for good, for those who are called according to His purpose" (Romans 8:28).

12 I Am Not "Fighting Cancer"!

Lesson Learned, Opportunity
Opened, or Purpose Pursued:

> I am NOT Fighting Cancer! Christ has Conquered It!

There was my name on a printed prayer list for a Christian ministry. It read, "Bill Bartlett—fighting cancer."

Something seemed wrong about that. I'm not fighting cancer. My doctors are. The drugs I am taking are. I depend on Christ for His sufficiency, power, and omnipotence over any-and-everything that may ever threaten me. And, if Jesus Christ, or even one of His angels, were to actually "fight" cancer, the "battle belongs to the Lord."

The victory has been won and will be won. I am a conqueror through Christ! I am joyfully leaning on Jesus as we together journey through this cancer treatment.

- "In all these things we are more than conquerors through Him Who loved us" (Rom. 8:37).
- "To me, to live is Christ and to die is gain" (Phil. 1:21).

13 All is OK

Lesson Learned, Opportunity Opened, or Purpose Pursued:

> Come What May, All is OK!

Fact: Jesus is gracious, loving, merciful, Lord and sovereign over all

Therefore, all is OK.

There is a human tendency for us to ask, "What if" God healed me?

Shouldn't the real Christian tendency be for us to say, "Even if..."? Consider the following two passages.

- As Shadrach, Meshach, and Abednego were about to be tossed into the fiery furnace, they said to Nebuchadnezzar,"If this be so, our God Whom we serve is able to deliver us from the burning fiery furnace, and He will deliver us out of your hand, O king. But if not, be it known to you, O king, that we will not serve your gods or worship the golden image that you have set up" (Dan. 3:17-18).

- "Though [read "<u>Even if...</u>"] the fig tree should not blossom, nor fruit be on the vines, the produce of the olive fail and the fields yield no food, the flock be cut off from the fold and there be no herd in the stalls, yet I will rejoice in the Lord; I will take joy in the God of my salvation" (Hab. 3:17-18).

Indeed, with Jesus, "Come what may, all is OK!"

14 A New Day (and Night) Job

Lesson Learned, Opportunity Opened, or Purpose Pursued:

> This Journey is My New Calling.

Over the forty years of my post-seminary life, I have had six "Calls":

1. Pastor of Christian Education and Youth, Arlington Hills Lutheran Church, St. Paul, Minnesota
2. Pastor Developer of a new mission church, Living Lord Lutheran Church, Bartlett, Illinois
3. Pastor of All Saints Lutheran Church, Phoenix, Arizona
4. Pastor of Lutheran Church of the Cross, Laguna Hills and Aliso Viejo, California
5. Founding Executive Director of Crean Lutheran High School, Irvine, California
6. Steward and Purveyor of Lessons, Opportunities, and Purposes Granted to a Cancer Patient Who Loves Jesus.

Each of these "Callings" required much from me. I was an evangelist, a preacher, a teacher, an administrator, an entrepreneur, prayer warrior, and a worship leader.

Yes, even in my last and current "Calling"—that of being a Christian cancer patient—I am given opportunities to fulfill each of these roles. As a matter of fact, this last "Calling," due to the 24/7 awareness—often in the middle of the night when I awaken from a "sweet dream" to the reality of being in cancer treatment—is all-consuming as I strive to "make the most of every opportunity" that this journey presents.

Jesus, please help me fulfill this Calling faithfully. I may have stepped away from my "day job" of my former "Calling," but I have stepped into a new job that is just as much of a holy Calling, and even more all-consuming! Amen.

15 You Are Not Your Own

Lesson Learned, Opportunity Opened, or Purpose Pursued:

"You Are Not Your Own; You Were Bought at a Price."
1 Corinthians 6:19-20

Patient-guilt.

Sure, we pay for our medical insurance. But, the amount of money that has been spent to keep me alive even up to the start of my enrollment in the clinical trial I'm now in far exceeds the total of all the medical insurance premiums we have ever paid—or ever will pay. That causes guilt.

Now add to this debt, that is far greater than I could ever pay, the additional costs of the research and expense of the experimental drug I take every two weeks, and one experiences "pile-on guilt"!

How can my life ever repay this debt? What can I do to repay the insurance company, or the medical and scientific community, for the investment they have made in me?

Dear Lord, Jesus, help me to live my life for others—all others—as the world has invested much in my medical care. And, dear Jesus, help me to live my life FOR YOU as You redeemed [bought] me at the price of Your own death on the Cross. I am NOT my own. I have been bought at a price. Let me please be a worthy investment, imbued with Your priceless redeeming grace, as I now live my life for You and others. Amen.

16 Proclaiming the Power of Christ From a Position of Weakness!

Lesson Learned, Opportunity Opened, or Purpose Pursued:

> This is a Unique and Challenging Calling.

While one of the blessings of immunotherapy is the lack of the severe toxic side effects of traditional chemotherapy, the most frequently cited side effect is tiredness. Sometimes, in my tired moments, I often reflect on the rigorous schedule that we had for decades. In those moments, I also pause to give thanks to the Lord for having given us the energy and the health to be able to persevere weeks on end without rest.

I now find myself in a new Calling—one of boldly, loudly, and as often as possible proclaiming the more-than-sufficient grace of Jesus Christ through difficult times. And, I find that I am doing this from a position of weakness and a lack of title or authority.

Before my diagnosis and treatment, while I was still employed in my prior Calling, I had a position, responsibilities, and a place in an org chart that enabled me to effect change and affect the direction of a corporation and many people's lives.

Enter cancer. Start treatment. End employment. Find myself not just lower on an org chart, but nowhere on an org chart. Accept a new Calling. Make the most of every opportunity— which suddenly seem more than I could imagine. Realize that people are listening. Accept the "mic" that is being handed to me by the Lord. Don't drop the mic, because the world is listening, and because everyone in the world will queue up in this line of human mortality at sometime, and they desperately want to know if indeed Jesus' grace is sufficient—even more than sufficient.

Such an opportunity and responsibility fuels me, motivates me, compels me, and encourages me to speak, proclaim, write, witness, and call attention to lessons that I have learned, opportunities that the Lord has opened, and purpose that the Lord has given to my life—even in and from this position of weakness.

17 Is This a Mountain Top Experience?

Lesson Learned, Opportunity Opened, or Purpose Pursued:

> This is a Mountain Top Holy Experience, not an Edge of the Cliff Threat.

In late 2014, after failed ABVD chemotherapy (each letter stands for a chemotherapy drug) for my Hodgkin's Lymphoma (90% of patients are cured through this treatment; I was in the 10% who were not cured), my oncologist told me we had another "second line" treatment—a stem cell transplant (SCT).

I asked about the approximate success rate of this SCT; my doctor replied, "50%." I asked what if I end up in the unsuccessful 50% category? He replied, "You are then at the edge of the cliff, with the rocks beginning to fall."

Hmmm. That was disconcerting to hear. And, imagine how I felt eight months later after a scan revealed that the cancer had returned even after the SCT.

But, by God's grace, research had progressed, during those months, to the point where, in March, 2015, several promising follow-up therapy options were available. One such option was a clinical trial using a new immunotherapy drug. Thanks be to the Lord and to ongoing research!

Let me now take you back to the discussion my oncologist and I had about being on the "edge of the cliff, with the rocks beginning to fall." When I first heard this, for some reason my mind went to the account of Moses standing on Mt. Nebo, overlooking the Promised Land (Deuteronomy 34), or Moses being on the mountain top with the Lord, resulting in Moses' face being radiant when he returned to the people because he had been talking with the Lord (Exodus 34:29).

It seems to me that we have a choice—are we "at the edge of the cliff" or are we "on Mt. Nebo" overlooking the Promised Land we are soon to enter? What a difference in perspective. One choice carries with it fear; the other choice is a mountain top experience, exuding and promising joy and homecoming.

Since my oncologist first mentioned that "edge of the cliff" comment, I have chosen the Holy Mountain Top, Mt. Nebo, perspective.

No fear; just joy and holy anticipation!

18 "Waiting for ~~Godot~~" ...God!

Lesson Learned, Opportunity Opened, or Purpose Pursued:

> I Feel Like I'm an Actor on Stage and "Waiting for ~~Godot~~" ...God! Lord, Help Me to Faithfully and Purposefully Wait for and Testify to You.

One of the strangest plays I've ever seen is "Waiting for Godot." What a portrayal of purposelessness, meaninglessness, and emptiness! Waiting, just putting in time, having meaningless conversations, occasional eruptions of despair, and clinging to false hope. How these words and phrases often describe human life—both those who are healthy as well as those who are suffering from diseases.

Contrast the sad quality and emptiness of life portrayed in this play with the purposeful, meaningful, joyous, highly anticipatory and full life of a disciple of Jesus who patiently, yet purposefully and enthusiastically, embraces each moment and each day while waiting for, and looking forward to, Christ's return! What a contrast!

Revelation 21:4 describes what is coming:

> "He will wipe away every tear from their eyes, and death shall be no more, neither shall there be mourning, nor crying, nor pain anymore, for the former things have passed away."

Lord Jesus, let me make the most of the stage-moment and microphone-moment this illness has given to me. Help me to glorify and witness to the sufficiency of Your grace and the joy of Your coming Kingdom!

"Amen. Come, Lord Jesus!" (Rev. 22:20).

19 Never Let it Get Old

Lesson Learned, Opportunity Opened, or Purpose Pursued:

> Never Let the Intensity or Exhilaration of this Journey Get Old! Keep Motivated! Keep Proclaiming! Don't Drop the Mic!

"I think it is right to refresh your memory as long as I live in the tent of this body, because I know that I will soon put it aside, as our Lord Jesus Christ has made clear to me. And I will make every effort to see that after my departure you will always be able to remember these things" (2 Peter 1:13-15).

During this time of cancer affliction and treatment, the microphone is in my hand, people are listening, the opportunity is present, and the purpose of this time is pregnant with possibilities!

Therefore, I am striving to …

- Make hay while the sun shines!
- Make the most of every opportunity!
- Strike while the iron is hot!
- Seize the day!
- Carpe diem!
- Not drop the mic!

This passage from 2 Peter 1 has been the motivation behind this list of "Lessons Learned, Opportunities Opened, and Purposes Pursued" as well as the following other projects to testify to Christ's sufficiency during this holy journey—not wanting to waste this suffering, but to redeem it with Kingdom purpose, and to make sure a legacy of trusting in the Lord is securely in place for our children, grandchildren, and others within my sphere of witness.

Therefore, I have been intentional about keeping busy and redeeming this time with Kingdom-related projects. These projects may be small building blocks, or even pebbles, in God's Kingdom/House, but I at least want to be a participant in His coming Kingdom—not one sidelined or sitting on the bench!

One of the most challenging and inspiring books I've ever read was written by two teenagers—Alex and Brett Harris, <u>Do Hard Things</u>. I selected this book for summer reading for Crean Lutheran High School a few years back. If two teenagers could do "hard things," then certainly I, being a grown adult with God-given experiences and relationships, need to do some "hard things"—at least harder than sitting passively in a hospital bed or in an infusion chair. So, I have committed to "stay on the field and not sit on the bench" during this time.

Here is a chronicled list of projects undertaken during my illness and treatment:

1. Began a list of "Lessons Learned" during this journey. August 2013.
2. Wrote a book, Divine Paradigm. October 2013-July 2014.
3. Made a video while in the hospital. Oct 2013.
4. Maintained a journal from diagnosis of recurrent Hodgkin's Lymphoma to 100 days post stem cell transplant. August 2014-February 2015.
5. Wrote an article about sufferings. December 2014.
6. Memorized at least two verses from each book of the Bible (to "hide in my heart" Psalm 119:11 and to "be prepared" 1 Peter 3:15 for when I may need them personally or for sharing). Memorized Romans 8. Lent 2014.
7. Started a "CANCER: Don't Drop the Mic!" blog. April 2015.
8. Made "be prepared" (I Peter 3:15) cards to hand out in appropriate situations such as with tips at restaurants, in

hotel rooms, and with fast food gift cards for homeless. May 2015.

9. Wrote an article about Student Debt: An Impoverished Education, highlighting the present student loan debt crisis and suggesting some solutions, written to help make Christian colleges and seminary education more affordable. September 2015.

10. Initiated a partnership between a well-respected, accredited Christian seminary and a new denomination that did not have a formal relationship with such a seminary for the purpose of providing a sustainable future of well-trained faithful pastors for this new denomination. November 2015 - July 2016.

11. Laid a foundation for and promoted a "Christian Worldview Seminar" (CWS) that could be taught as an early college course for credit by a Christian university, targeting public high school students. The CWS would be two 3-credit courses spread out over the junior and senior year, instilling Christian worldview, Christian critical thinking, and Christian values as part of the undergirding of Christian formation and lifelong discipleship. March 2016

12. This project! September 2013 - August 2016.

What next, Lord? I'm ready!

20 No Self-Justification Needed

Lesson Learned, Opportunity Opened, or Purpose Pursued:

I Do Not Need to Self-Justify My Existence or Life or Try to Make Excuses for My Life to Continue.

This "learning" is placed directly beneath the above "learning" which listed projects I have undertaken to redeem or vindicate this time impacted by cancer and treatment and to make the most of every opportunity to proclaim Jesus Christ, His grace, and His coming Kingdom. (Don't Drop the Mic!)

This post was prompted by an Advent devotion Cindy and I read last evening. The devotion was in "The Dawning of Indestructible Joy" by John Piper. While reading the devotion, it dawned (an insightful naming of Piper's devotion) on me that the aforementioned litany could appear to be a self-justification of my existence now that I am not gainfully employed and a bit "sidelined" due to my cancer treatment.

Piper's devotion did a great job of revealing the "upside-down" nature of our Lord's values. Our achievements are to be done "unto Him" (Colossians 3:23-24) and for "His glory" (Isaiah 43:7)—not done to justify, elevate, or promote ourselves.

Whatever we do, in word or deed—or whatever we don't, or cannot, or fail to do—we still do all only unto Him, giving thanks to God the Father through Christ.

Our deeds or accomplishments are only expressions of our praise to our Lord Jesus—something we were created to do no matter what we do or don't do.

Perhaps my Calling now is to better understand that ALL of my life—my productive, employed life, as well as my "patient" life—is simply to just "praise and thank the Lord."

21 Stand Up!

Lesson Learned, Opportunity Opened, or Purpose Pursued:

> "Stand up! What are You Doing Down on your Face?"
> Joshua 7:10

Once in a while, I feel tired. Really tired. So-tired-that-I-cannot-roll-over-in-bed tired. During those times, I try to sleep. If I cannot sleep but find that I am still so-tired-that-I-cannot-roll-over, then I try to use that time as "bonus prayer time." I rehearse Scripture memory verses or passages, and I pray.

There are other times when I am figuratively "face down"—tempted to give up, to have a pity party, to throw in the towel, or turn in my uniform.

This is the context into which Joshua 7:10 speaks—or shouts!

> The Lord said to Joshua, "Stand up! What are you doing down on your face?" Joshua 7:10.

I love this verse. And, I need to hear and heed this verse on occasion. Sometimes, I get down—like Joshua—from self-pity. The Lord has no time for this. He can—and does—use people from positions of weakness, sickness, and lack of resources. As a matter of fact, it is often in those moments that He hands us a microphone and says, "The world is listening. What are you going to say?"

In those moments, stand tall. Speak boldly. Don't Drop the Mic!

> "Be on your guard; stand firm in the faith; be courageous; be strong" (1 Cor. 16:13).

22 God's Word as Medicine

Lesson Learned, Opportunity Opened, or Purpose Pursued:

> Memory Verses are Good Medicine.

During my treatment, thus far, I've had much medicine infused into my body: many variations of toxic chemotherapy and lots of antibiotics, saline, heparin, blood, platelets, and more.

God's Word has also been pumped in—with a promised long-term, efficacious, and healing potency! I read the Bible daily just as I receive medication and drugs because I need the treating and healing power they all provide. Never would I say to my doctor, "No thanks on the immunotherapy today; I'm too busy." In the same way, how dare we ever say to our Lord, "No thanks, Lord, on Your Word today; I'm fine without it." Wrong! Dangerous! Arrogant! Stupid!

In addition to reading God's Word, memorizing God's Word provides a wonderful reservoir of power, peace, and promise from our Lord Jesus. Both my wife and I have committed much Scripture to memory in order to call upon it when we are in need.

Memory verses are a great comfort, bringing comfort at night, during treatment, in the recovery room, and at any moment a visitor, despair or fear knocks.

- "I have hidden Your Word in my heart…" (Psalm 119:11a).
- Also, God promises that His Word will "… accomplish what I desire and achieve the purpose for which I sent it" (Isaiah 55:11).

23 Acrostics

Lesson Learned, Opportunity Opened, or Purpose Pursued:

> Grace is "G-od's R-iches A-t C-hrist's E-xpense"

I've always loved acrostics. They are good memory tools, and they are useful in providing a structure for teaching or reminding us of a truth. Over the years (decades!), I've collected and created some acrostics which teach valuable messages of the Gospel.

Here are my "Top Ten Acrostics":

1. Cross (Christ redeems our sinful selves)
2. Grace (God's riches at Christ's expense)
3. Faith (forsaking all I trust Him), cross (Christ redeems our sinful selves)
4. Hope (His omnipotent promises everlasting)
5. INRI (the inscription, meaning "Jesus of Nazareth King of the Jews," above Christ on the cross; as an acrostic: I need redemption immediately)
6. Pray (an excellent order or framework for our prayers—praise, repent, ask, yield)
7. Self (sinners excuse large faults)
8. Sinner (self-intoxicated narcissist never expressing repentance)
9. Saints (sinners are invited near the Savior—what Gospel that is!)
10. Disciples (do I serve Christ in persevering love evidencing sanctification?)

Each of the phrases in the above acrostics conveys a fuller meaning of the word itself. I have used all of the above acrostics in teaching, preaching, and daily witnessing opportunities—as well as personal devotion and encouragement when I am in need of the Gospel message.

I invite you to use them as well—and to create and share some of your own acrostics which are helpful in passing on the saving G.R.A.C.E. of Jesus. After all, we are His D.I.S.C.I.P.L.E.S.!

24 How Can This be Bad?

Lesson Learned, Opportunity Opened, or Purpose Pursued:

> Going to Be With Jesus is NOT a Bad Thing; It is a Good Thing!

I once heard a story about a little girl who, with her parents, was taking a trip to see Grandma. Grandma lived in another state, so they were on their way to an airport to catch their flight. The mother was always a little frightened about flying. And, the little girl had never been in an airplane before—and knew that the plane flew miles high in the sky. Yet, the little girl went skipping and hopping down the concourse of the airport. The mother asked the little girl, "How can you be so full of joy? Aren't you afraid of flying in the airplane?" The little girl, overflowing with joy, replied, "How can I be afraid; we're going to Grandma's!"

Going to be with Jesus is not a bad thing; it is a good thing! Without sounding oddly morbid or inappropriate, shouldn't we all be skipping and hopping with joy at the prospect of "going to Jesus"?

This means that, at some time, we are all going to die—unless Christ comes first. And, we are all in the same mortal line, never knowing our true place in that line as we daily find our places in that line changing. So, whether we are still on "this side" or if we have arrived in Heaven, there is the joy of "being with Jesus" that calms our fears, fuels our joy, and takes away the sting of death!

"Death is not banishment; it is a return from exile" (Charles Spurgeon, Morning Devotions, April 20).

- "Behold! I tell you a mystery. We shall not all sleep, but we shall all be changed, 52 in a moment, in the twinkling of an eye, at the last trumpet. For the trumpet will sound, and the dead will be raised imperishable, and we shall be changed. 53 For this perishable body must put on the imperishable, and this mortal body must put on immortality. 54 When the perishable puts on the imperishable, and the mortal puts on immortality, then shall come to pass the saying that is written: "Death is swallowed up in victory." 55"O death, where is your victory? O death, where is your sting?" 56 The sting of death is sin, and the power of sin is the law. 57 But thanks be to God, who gives us the victory through our Lord Jesus Christ" (1 Cor 15:51-57).

- "For to me to live is Christ, and to die is gain. 22 If I am to live in the flesh, that means fruitful labor for me. Yet which I shall choose I cannot tell. 23 I am hard pressed between the two. My desire is to depart and be with Christ, for that is far better. 24 But to remain in the flesh is more necessary on your account" (Phil. 1:21-24).

25 "Amen. Come, Lord Jesus"

Lesson Learned, Opportunity
Opened, or Purpose Pursued:

> What is Death to the Christian Other Than an Early
> Coming of Christ?

The last prayer of the Bible is found in Revelation 22:20,

> "Amen. Come, Lord Jesus."

What is death to the Christian, but an early coming of Jesus and a glorious answer to the last prayer of the Bible, "Amen. Come, Lord Jesus"?

We don't pray, "Come, Lord Jesus; but not now!" Rather, we pray for, yearn for, and look forward to our Lord's response to this final prayer as He will come again—either at the end of all human history or at the time of our passing to be with the Lord in Heaven forever.

Amen. Come, Lord Jesus! Please come soon!

26 Your Final Answer!

Lesson Learned, Opportunity Opened, or Purpose Pursued:

> "What will I Answer on that Day When an Account is Demanded of Me, How I Spent the Whole Time of Life That was Given to me Down to My Last Moment? … Is there yet One upon Whom I can call? It is Jesus."
> -St. Anselm

I am a collector of quotes. One of the quotes that is among my top five favorites is from St. Anselm, a Christian theologian and writer from the 11th and 12th centuries.

I love this quote! As a matter of fact, I have let my family know that I want this read at my memorial service. It is a clear proclamation of trust and faith in Jesus. And, it is my final plea before seeing Jesus face to face!

> "What will I answer on that Day when an account is demanded of me, how I spent the whole time of life that was given to me down to my last moment?
>
> O dread! Have I have trusted in the one true God? Or, have I looked to idols or lesser spirits? Have I accepted Jesus as my living Lord and Savior? Or, have I only observed Him from afar as a distant figure?
>
> O Lord, You alone are Holy. You alone are righteous. O the dread of my sinfulness before Your holiness.
>
> Your Kingly Holiness and Righteousness demand what we cannot give.
>
> On this side there will be the accusing sins, on that side terrifying justice;
>
> Below appears the horrid chaos of hell, above the Holy

and Righteous Judge;

Inside, the burning conscience, outside, the burning world.

If one were righteous, one might be saved. But, alas, no one is righteous.

Where, then, shall the sinner, thus caught, hide?

To hide will be impossible, to appear intolerable.

Where can I flee? What is my plea? Where is salvation?

Is there yet One upon Whom I can call? Is there yet grace that calms my soul?

It is Jesus… Jesus the Righteous Who on the Cross bled for me and bore my sin and the sin of the world.

Jesus is the One upon Whom I call. He alone is my Risen Savior, my Redeemer, my Lord, my door to eternal life.

Revive, sinner; do not despair. Hope in Him; flee to Him.

Therefore, Jesus, be Thou my Savior for Thy Name's sake. Thy mercy overcomes every offense. Thy grace opens Heaven's door."

　　　　　　　　　--St. Anselm of Canterbury,
1033-1109 AD, paraphrase

27 In Christ

Lesson Learned, Opportunity Opened, or Purpose Pursued:

> In Christ (... the Best, Safest, and Most Joyful Place to Be)!

"In Christ." What a glorious thought! What an answer to prayer! What a safe place to be! What a joyful place to be! It is the BEST place to be now, tomorrow, and forever!

"In Christ" is a Biblical phrase. It is a positional phrase. It is a destination phrase. It is a representative or familial phrase. To be "in Christ" is our prayer, our passion, our gift of grace, and the result of Christ's death and resurrection.

This journey has given me a new appreciation of being "in Christ"—the best, safest, most joyful, and eternal place to be.

The closing that I most frequently use when writing a letter or email is ...

> In Christ (...the best, safest, and most joyful place to be!), Bill Bartlett

My prayer for you is that you are also "in Christ." It IS the best, safest, and most joyful place to be!

28 The Pearl of Great Price ... the One Thing Necessary!

Lesson Learned, Opportunity Opened, or Purpose Pursued:

"Whatever Lacks the Name of Jesus Cannot Completely Win Me, However Well Expressed, Polished, and True-Appearing."- Cicero

A couple of chapters ago, I mentioned that I am a collector of quotes. My all-time favorite, single, cherished non-Biblical quote is by another Christian Saint, theologian and writer St. Augustine, 354-430 AD.

After his conversion to Christianity, Augustine, after reading one of his favorite pre-Christian authors, Cicero (who wrote in the 2nd century BC), lamented:

> "The only thing to dim my enthusiasm is the fact that the name of Christ was not there...for by this name, by Your mercy, O Lord, this name of my Savior, Your Son, is my life given. Therefore, whatever lacks this Name cannot completely win me, however well expressed, polished, and true-appearing."

This quote expresses the preeminence of Jesus above all else. This quote also calls attention to, and makes us sensitive to, moments, endeavors, or gatherings which do not include the presence and acknowledgment of Jesus Christ.

This is at the heart of what I have called "Jesus-proofing" in the churches and schools in which I have served. If a room, or a sermon, or Bible study, or a letter, or a memo, or a conversation does not contain Jesus (in word, picture, or reference), then that entity or communication or effort is lacking "however well expressed, polished, and true-appearing" it may otherwise be.

Bible passages support this contention by St. Augustine:

- "The kingdom of heaven is like a merchant in search of fine pearls, who, on finding one pearl of great value, went and sold all that he had and bought it" (Matt. 13:45-46).

- "Now as they went on their way, Jesus entered a village. And a woman named Martha welcomed Him into her house. 39 And she had a sister called Mary, who sat at the Lord's feet and listened to his teaching. 40 But Martha was distracted with much serving. And she went up to Him and said, "Lord, do you not care that my sister has left me to serve alone? Tell her then to help me." 41 But the Lord answered her, "Martha, Martha, you are anxious and troubled about many things, 42 but one thing is necessary. Mary has chosen the good portion, which will not be taken away from her" (Luke 10:38-42).

Treatment, comfort, peace, and even healing are all ultimately lacking if they ignore the name and person of Christ!

29 Alleluia Anyhow!

Lesson Learned, Opportunity Opened, or Purpose Pursued:

> When the Darkness Closes in, Lord, Still I Will Say, "Blessed be the Name of the Lord!"

A mark of growing discipleship in Christ is the ability to say, "Alleluia anyhow"—and mean it!

How easy it is to be a fair weather disciple of Jesus Christ, announcing alleluias in the midst of affluence and smooth sailing.

How refining it is to resolutely say, "Alleluia anyhow!" when enduring difficulties, illness, and tragedy.

There is a blessing to be cherished in being firm in one's faith in times of trouble. Why? Because Jesus is Lord, sovereign Ruler, King of kings, and Savior of my soul whether I am in calm waters or stormy seas.

One of my favorite "Alleluia anyhow" Bible passages that speaks directly to this is Habakkuk 3:17-18,

> "Though the fig tree should not blossom, nor fruit be on the vines, the produce of the olive fail and the fields yield no food, the flock be cut off from the fold and there be no herd in the stalls, yet I will rejoice in the Lord; I will take joy in the God of my salvation."

During this journey, I have particularly enjoyed—and have been ministered to—by three great Christian songs of truth and encouragement. All three of these songs are wonderful variations on the theme, "Alleluia anyhow!" I invite you to listen to the songs and join the chorus in singing, "Alleluia anyhow!"

Blessed be Your Name

(Lyrics—Beth and Matt Redman)
http://www.godtube.com/watch/?v=02M20FNU

(10,000 Reasons) Bless the Lord
(Lyrics—Matt Redman and Jonas Myrin)
http://www.godtube.com/watch/?v=WLPKDWNX

Trust in you
(Lyrics—Lauren Daigle, Mabury and Michael Farren)
http://www.godtube.com/watch/?v=0CBBEJNU

30 Hope vs. Certainty

Lesson Learned, Opportunity Opened, or Purpose Pursued:

> True Biblical Hope is Certainty, Not Wishful Thinking!

The certainty of resurrection to eternal life through Christ is more than "hope" as hope is commonly understood in our modern language.

The Greek word for hope is "elpis" and it means "waiting for something that is certain and that will come to pass in the future." It is more like anticipation rather than hoping for something that just "may" happen.

Our current English language has corrupted this original meaning of this wonderful word. Today, we "hope" to win the lottery (while knowing we won't), we "hope" our favorite NFL team will win the Super Bowl (while knowing they probably won't), and we "hope" that next year will be better than this year (while not having any hard data or evidence that it will).

Contrast that current-English-usage definition of "hope" with Biblical, elpis-defined "hope." We hope that Jesus is coming again (He will!), we hope that Jesus' shed blood on the Cross is sufficient to cover all my sins (it is!), and we "hope" that Heaven will be better than earth (it will!).

The Biblical meaning of hope, therefore, is certainty of what is coming, not a "fat chance" that something may go our way.

- Hebrews 11:1, "faith is the <u>assurance</u> of things hoped for...."
- Job said it well in 19:25, "I <u>know</u> that my Redeemer lives."

Christian "hope" is certainty—not yet here, but surely coming! What holy anticipation and joy that is!

31 Deceiving Outward Appearances

Lesson Learned, Opportunity Opened, or Purpose Pursued:

No Matter How Healthy One Looks, Our Human Bodies are Not Long for This World.

I feel great and, outwardly, even look healthy—in spite of the fact that I am in a clinical trial with an experimental cancer treatment.

There were times during my earlier (and unsuccessful) treatments for cancer when I did not look healthy or vital! In the midst of high dose chemotherapy just before a stem cell transplant, I looked like a pale, puffed up (due to medicine) Pillsbury Doughboy. But, now, at least for a season, I look pretty healthy. The immunotherapy I am receiving during the clinical trial in which I am enrolled is not toxic like chemotherapy or physically abusive to a body like surgery or radiation can be.

But, what a deceiving message my outward appearance gives! I am being treated for recurrent cancer, for Heaven's sake! I'm in a clinical trial because approved therapies don't work!

What an allegory of life. No matter our outer appearance or our inner physical health, we all are mortal (meaning we will die) heading toward either eternal life or death, no matter if we are diagnosed with an illness or not. Our eternal home is in Heaven with Christ, not here in this mortal life.

Jesus chastised the Pharisees who made an art of looking fine on the outside but being as good as dead on the inside:

> "Woe to you, scribes and Pharisees, hypocrites! For you clean the outside of the cup and the plate, but inside they are full of greed and self-indulgence. 26 You blind Pharisee! First clean the inside of the cup and the plate,

that the outside also may be clean. Woe to you, scribes and Pharisees, hypocrites! For you are like whitewashed tombs, which outwardly appear beautiful, but within are full of dead people's bones and all uncleanness. 28 So you also outwardly appear righteous to others, but within you are full of hypocrisy and lawlessness" (Matt. 23: 25-28).

How shallow are most of our encounters with others! Now, I am not saying that deep within every outwardly fine-looking person is a Pharisaical hypocrite. But, I guess I am saying is that inside every person, no matter the outward appearance of healthy and happy, or gaunt and ill, there is a sinner, like me, in need of what only Jesus can give.

Perhaps we should look at all people, including ourselves—no matter the outer appearance—as eternal beings headed toward eternal life or death. What a perspective change that would be. What a contrast compared to how the world looks at outward appearances. Rather than looking at only the outward appearance of people, or even rather than looking for the hidden sins and faults inside others, perhaps we should strive to look for, see, and seek Christ "in" others—and do what we can to encourage a living Christ within every person.

To be concerned about the eternal destiny of every person, rather than being concerned about how others—or we—appear outwardly would deepen relationships, invite greater transparency, and redefine our perspective and definition of beauty and worth. To be concerned about the eternal destiny of every person—which means that we would be concerned above all else with each person's relationship to Jesus—would result in a new appreciation of beauty and life that would make the results of the most opaque cataract surgery pale in comparison.

Just as we cannot judge a book by its cover, nor can we or should we ever imagine that we can know what is going on within a person based on outer appearances. Let us commit to seeing the person within—the person for whom Jesus died. And, let us be most concerned about displaying, even radiating, the most beautiful, handsome, and compelling feature that best defines and presents us—Christ in us, the hope of glory (Col. 1:27).

32 Eternal Optimism

Lesson Learned, Opportunity
Opened, or Purpose Pursued:

> Christ in You, the Hope (elpis, certainty!) of Glory!
> Colossians 1:27

Colossians 1:27, "The glorious riches of this mystery... is Christ in you, the hope [certainty!] of glory."

Cancer may be in my body, but so is Jesus Christ. And, the battle has been won.

> "I am convinced that neither death nor life, neither angels nor demons, neither the present nor the future, nor any powers, neither height nor depth, nor anything else in all creation [including cancer], will be able to separate us from the love of God that is in Christ Jesus our Lord" (Romans 8:39).

And, remember from a previous chapter, "hope," in Greek ("elpis"), means not wishful fantasy, but simply waiting for what is assured and certain.

No matter what, the glory of the presence of Christ is a given for those who love Jesus.

33 Unlimited Power Source

Lesson Learned, Opportunity Opened, or Purpose Pursued:

> When I Cannot, Jesus Can!

When my energy lags, Christ provides.

I love the message from Colossians 1:29, "To this end I labor [proclaiming Christ in word and deed], striving (agōnizomai) with all His energy (energeia) that works so powerfully within me."

There are two words which are most important to me in this verse:

- agōnizomai
- energeia

Mine is the agōnizomai—striving to the point of the root of that word, agonizing pursuit and labor.

Christ's is the energeia—the power, the energy, and the strength beyond my energy that enables, powers, and carries me through what I, without Christ, would not be able to do!

34 The Blessed Joy of a Blog or Journal

Lesson Learned, Opportunity Opened, or Purpose Pursued:

A Blog or a Journal is Good Therapy and a Good Practice.

In August of 2013, I started this journaling project, keeping track of "Lessons Learned, Opportunities Opened, and Purposes Pursued," as a means of helping me to keep focused on Christ, attentive to what the Lord is teaching me through this journey, and as a possible means of helping others who are also, or will be, on this cancer treatment trail.

The journal entries follow no particular theme or sequence. Rather, they are simply learnings, opportunities, or a purpose that the journey or the Lord reveals to me as I take one day at a time.

Each entry is made with a prayer that I will ...

- Never, ever forget the "Lesson Learned"—even if, by the grace of God, I am "cured" of cancer;
- Always and ever take advantage of "Opportunities Opened" through this journey—opportunities which, without cancer, would not have opened;
- With a vengeance and tenacity reflective of Jesus and His grace, pursue the purpose of our lives—which is to glorify the Lord by being a faithful steward of the life our Lord gives us;
- And never, ever "Drop the Mic" for the rest of my life as I use all these experiences, learnings, opportunities, and purpose to the praise of our Lord's glory—which is the mission of my life (and every life).

By writing this journal and by maintaining a blog for the above purposes, I tether myself to an intentional act of letting these experiences, learnings, opportunities, and purpose steer my life—and, prayerfully, shedding some light on the paths of others who travel similar journeys.

This is, for me, good therapy and a good practice.

35 Not in Vain!

Lesson Learned, Opportunity Opened, or Purpose Pursued:

My Labor in the Lord is Never in Vain—Ever!

How important it is to remain purposeful, useful, and busy throughout our lives—and especially, for me, during this time.

I Corinthians 15:58 is a great verse of encouragement for me,

> "Therefore, my dear brothers and sisters, stand firm.
> Let nothing move you. Always give yourselves fully to
> the work of the Lord, because you know that your labor
> in the Lord is not in vain."

So much of my life—and identity—was tied up in what I was doing in my Calling as founding director of Crean Lutheran High School that when I stepped away from this ministry, I immediately felt a vacuum.

My productivity—at least to me—seemed to stop.

At first, this depressed me. But then, I realized that a new Calling was surfacing—responding to the opportunities the Lord was setting before me every day. My new goal and passion were to be a faithful "steward of opportunities." And, the Lord has not slowed His offerings of opportunities that He sets before me every day!

Some of these opportunities seem to fit into a regular and recurring pattern: there are always people to pray for, emails of encouragement to write, and little things I can do for others and the Lord's Kingdom.

Some opportunities are unique and something that I would never, previously, even thought of or had time to pursue.

Some opportunities could be defined as "hard things"—things that required lots of focus, energy, and effort.

All of these opportunities are gifts from our Lord—given to me during a time in life when I am weakened by illness, but strengthened by His grace, for the great and precious purpose of "laboring" for the Lord—and all the while knowing and finding joy in the fact and promise that "my labor in the Lord is never in vain"!

36 Living Above Bad News

Lesson Learned, Opportunity Opened, or Purpose Pursued:

> There is Holy Anticipation Even in the Midst of Bad News.

This journey is teaching me much. Yesterday and today, I learned a lesson about keeping an eternal perspective and not getting too depressed about setbacks.

The lesson deals with a Christian response to bad news. Hmmm… yesterday (May 2015), my doctor called and told me I did not qualify for the clinical trial which would give me access to a new, promising immunotherapy drug, Opdivo.

That was a hard and disappointing phone call. My doctor had previously indicated that my condition was approaching the "edge of the cliff" stage, but yet he also indicated that there were new promising treatments coming down the pipeline of research.

The lesson I learned was that, even in the midst of disappointment—or perhaps better stated, ESPECIALLY in the midst of disappointment, for the Christian, there is always the holy and joyous anticipation that comes with the prayer and cry, "What now, Lord?" as we then wait confidently for His more than sufficient grace and power.

God is good … all the time. All the time … God is good.

Because of this, we can always be of good cheer and be full of optimism as we wait for our Lord to open new doors—even if it is Heaven's door!

37 Undulations

Lesson Learned, Opportunity Opened, or Purpose Pursued:

> For the Christian, What Goes Down Must Come Up!

C.S. Lewis, in his book, <u>The Screwtape Letters</u>, writes about "undulations" in one of his chapters—the extreme ups and downs, peaks and valleys, like waves, of life.

Screwtape, the chief devil, instructing Wormwood, one of his understudy devils, on the art of luring a "patient" (a human) to hell, warned Wormwood of the dangers of undulations:

> "Our cause is never more in danger than when a human, no longer desiring, but still intending, to do our Enemy's will, looks round upon a universe from which every trace of Him seems to have vanished, and asks why he has been forsaken, and still obeys." -C.S. Lewis, <u>The Screwtape Letters.</u>

Two days ago, with news of not qualifying for a clinical trial was a tough *trough* day. Today, I received news that I was accepted into the clinical trial—a peak day.

Lessons to be learned:

- Perseverance in trusting the Lord will get us through life's storms to Heaven's shore.
- Anticipate the Lord's goodness and grace at ALL times.
- God is good … all the time. All the time … God is good!
- Indeed, how wonderful, wonderful, wonderful it is that we can say "Praise the Lord because or for..." (during peaks) and "Alleluia anyhow..." (during valleys) with equal enthusiasm, confidence, trust, anticipation, and joy!

38 The Mist Will Rise

Lesson Learned, Opportunity Opened, or Purpose Pursued:

> Even 97 Years is a Brief Mist!

In a Billy Graham devotional, Dr. Graham reflected on his "biggest surprise of life." He said that it was the brevity of earthly life. Remember, as of the writing of this chapter, Dr. Graham is 97 years old. Yet, he calls this "brevity"!

Dr. Graham could speak this way because the perspective of his life is measured against eternity.

> "With the Lord, one day is as a thousand years, and a thousand years as one day" (2 Peter 3:8).

The real focus and wonder in our lives shouldn't be on the brevity of earthly life, but rather on the length and joy of eternal life through Jesus.

> "What is your life? You are a mist that appears for a little while and then vanishes" (James 4:14).

Whenever we are in the midst of an illness, a hurdle, a difficulty, or a suffering, we can remember, "This too will pass."

What then will last?

In my childhood home, there was a small needlepoint, framed artwork, about four inches by six inches, that I saw every day. Based on a passage from 1 Corinthians 3:11-15, it read,

> "Just one life will soon be past. Only what's done for Christ will last."

What's the encouragement in all this? What is the lesson then to be learned in this message? Billy Graham again speaks the answer in one of his famous quotes:

> "Only three things last forever: The Lord, His Word, and His people."

Hold on to what is eternal. That is Jesus, His Word, and His people. Everything else—even the cancer—is a mist!

39 Perseverance

Lesson Learned, Opportunity Opened, or Purpose Pursued:

> This is but a Light and Momentary Trouble!

Perspective makes a difference. Perseverance makes a difference. When both work together, our illnesses, pains, treatments, and threats become but "light and momentary troubles."

I love the following two passages:

- "I consider that our present sufferings are not worth comparing with the glory that will be revealed in us" (Rom. 8:18).
- "Therefore we do not lose heart. Though outwardly we are wasting away, yet inwardly we are being renewed day by day. For our light and momentary troubles are achieving for us an eternal glory that far outweighs them all...For we know that if the earthly tent we live in is destroyed, we have a building from God, an eternal house in heaven, not built by human hands" (2 Cor. 4:16-17, 5:1).

As I age and find my former strength "washing away," and as I recognize the frailty of my human flesh, I find comfort in the inverse relationship that the above passage describes between my "earthly tent" and my "eternal house in heaven" (my resurrection body). As my body, strength, athleticism, etc., "waste away," my "eternal house in heaven" (my resurrection body) is being prepared and strengthened.

In the perspective of eternity, even the most uncomfortable and debilitating result of and treatment for illnesses or disabilities are but "light and momentary troubles" that will soon be over and forgotten as we will revel and rejoice in our resurrection bodies!

40 Living in the Exciting Present With Jesus

Lesson Learned, Opportunity Opened, or Purpose Pursued:

Moment by Moment Dependence on the Lord!

It is an odd—but holy—feeling to be on an "experimental drug," knowing that even the doctors do not have a clear vision of how or if the medicine will work.

This creates a "daily awareness of the gift of this moment" and a "daily readiness" for departing this life and being with the Lord.

This is a good thing, even a blessing.

In Spurgeon's daily devotion for July 16 (morn), we are reminded:

> "This hourly dependence our Lord is determined that we shall feel and recognize, for He only permits us to pray for "daily bread," and only promises that "as our days our strength shall be." Is it not best for us that it should be so, that we may often repair to his throne, and constantly be reminded of his love?"

Let us together resolve to cherish and depend on the constant, hour by hour, day by day sufficient grace of our Lord Jesus— in good times and in bad times, in good health and in times of treatment! How exciting it is to live in this absolute moment-by-moment dependence on our Lord Jesus!

41 Holy Words

Lesson Learned, Opportunity Opened, or Purpose Pursued:

> The Power of the WORD!

"In the beginning was the Word…" (John 1:1).

Words are powerful! God created all that exists through a Word. Jesus is the Word incarnate. Even our words are powerful. They conjure up feelings of love, gratitude, fear, or anxiety. Therefore, we should choose our words—words spoken, words contemplated, words read, words written—carefully.

I love certain words and often reflect on and use individual words like a needle on a compass—to guide my thoughts and life. Here are a few words I consider holy and instructive for my life.

1. Hope: From the Greek. "elpis," meaning "anticipating a certainty"—not just a blind hope!

2. Priorities: How important it is to moment by moment sort and then focus on, in sorted order, tasks, thoughts, projects, and Ultimate Concerns.

3. Focus: The world is full of distractions. There is an art to maintaining focus on the Lord and Kingdom matters in the midst of the siren calls of the world all around us.

4. Today: Today is a gift from our Lord. How we too often taint the gift of today from our Lord by bringing in regrets from yesterday, or worries about tomorrow.

5. Jesus: Jesus is the holiest of words. Jesus is the personal name of our personal Savior. There is power in the name of Jesus because His name, like a prayer, invokes His presence and blessings.

6. Grace: As an acrostic, this word reminds us that we have "God's Riches At Christ's Expense." It is by grace that we are saved.

7. Redeemed: We are doubly owned by our Lord. He created us. Then, He bought us back from our lost-in-sin state through the death and resurrection of Jesus. The word redeemed brings to mind God's love in creating us, and His love in buying us back (redemption) through His Son.

8. Sufficient: What a wonderful word that reminds us that "Jesus only" is all we need. He is all powerful! He is all loving. He is able. He is with us—Immanuel.

9. Joy: Jesus came that our joy may be full (John 15:11). What a wonderful Savior—not just a Savior Who saves us for Himself, but a Savior Who saves us to have joy and life to the full!

10. Grateful: Given all that our Lord Jesus does for us, how can we keep from overflowing with gratitude every day?

11. Purpose: We were created for his glory (Isaiah 43:7)—that's purpose. We were created as our Lord's masterpieces or handiwork for good works prepared in advance for us to do (Ephesians 2:10)—that's purpose.

12. Strive: From the Greek, "agon," (related to our English word, "agony") which means hard effort—fueled by our Lord's energy working within us (Colossians 1.29)!

42 A Different Point of View

Lesson Learned, Opportunity Opened, or Purpose Pursued:

"From Now On…" I Have a Different "Point of View"!

"From now on we regard no one [or anything—even illnesses] from a worldly point of view" (2 Cor. 5:16).

Events often change us. Cancer changes us. "From now on…" describes my life after diagnosis of cancer. My life is different. "From now on…" my life is different because cancer has given me a new point of view. It is no longer a worldly point of view. From now on, my perspective on the world, the lens through which I see the world, others, myself, life's purpose, and creation itself, is not just filtered by, but focused on, Jesus Christ.

"From now on…," because of cancer, the "point of view" by which I sense and see and relate to anyone and everything is transformed to the degree that my whole life and being now order everything in relationship to Jesus Christ.

- I will cherish every day as a gift from the Lord. I will not take good health, or even days when I feel good, for granted, but will live my life in thankfulness to the Lord, the giver of life, every day.
- I will be more sensitive to others because I know that all others suffer in some way, and that Jesus is sufficient for all suffering.
- I will appreciate the medical community—from scientists who discover new and effective treatments, to doctors and nurses who treat the sick, to aides who give TLC to patients in hospitals and treatment centers—and let them know of my gratitude every chance I have.

This means instead of focusing on being sick, I celebrate that I am under the daily care of the Great Physician.

Instead of focusing on suffering, I focus on God's comfort.

Instead of worrying about what the future holds, I joyfully anticipate that Christ holds my present as well as my future.

Instead of despairing about death, I rejoice in the life that Jesus gives.

From now on, this is my new point of view.

43 For the Lord!

Lesson Learned, Opportunity Opened, or Purpose Pursued:

"For the Lord..." is Our Purpose, Our Charge, and Our Joy!

"If we live, we live for the Lord; and if we die, we die for the Lord. So, whether we live or die, we belong to the Lord" (Rom. 14:8).

"For the Lord" is a purposeful statement. It conveys the direction of our lives, the conviction of our lives, the goal of our lives, and the allegiance of our lives.

"For the Lord" is like a battle-cry as we march against cancer or other illnesses or struggles.

"For the Lord" is an expression of our grateful hearts, as we live or die "for the Lord" Who lived and died for our forgiveness, life, and eternal salvation.

44 God's Timing

Lesson Learned, Opportunity Opened, or Purpose Pursued:

God's Timing is Not Our Timing!

Our Lord's timing is better than our understanding.

My original diagnosis of Hodgkin's Lymphoma was a long process, taking almost two months and causing us, back then, to be very impatient.

Then, the first two lines of treatment failed—both traditional ABVD chemotherapy (which usually is 90% successful) and the stem cell transplant (which is about 50% successful after ABVD failure).

If the diagnosis had been quicker, or if I had not undergone the first two lines of treatment, taking eighteen months and giving me the necessary treatment qualifications, the Clinical Trial of Opdivo would not have been available when I was in need.

The Clinical Trial just became available in December 2014. Only a few months earlier, my oncologist said that we were on our last treatment option. But, the delay kept me alive and made me a candidate for this new Clinical Trial—and even for other new treatments yet to come on the market that were not previously available.

Praise the Lord—in all circumstances ... we simply cannot see the whole picture, but we do see Jesus.

> "...when Jesus heard that Lazarus was sick, He stayed where He was two more days..." (John 11:6).

> "We know that in all things God works for the good of those who love Him, who have been called according to His purpose" (Rom. 8:28).

"The Lord is not slow to fulfill his promise [of coming again] as some count slowness, but is patient toward you, not wishing that any should perish, but that all should reach repentance" (2 Peter 3:9).

His timing is full of grace.

45 Today!

Lesson Learned, Opportunity Opened, or Purpose Pursued:

> Each Day, Isolated in Itself in Terms of Time, but Received as a Gift from the Lord, is a Holy Entity, which can be as Full of Joy, Even While Having Cancer, as the Happiest and Most Joy-Filled Day that You or Anyone Has Ever Had.

The above sentence hit me like a ton of bricks one day. I was in the hospital, just after my stem cell transplant, still in isolation, but feeling pretty good and for some reason overflowing with a sense of gratitude for life and all the doctors, nurses, and care that I had received and continued to receive, and with an affection for my family, including all the memories I had, and hoped for memories yet to be made.

In that context, the above thought came to mind. I felt that I, in that day, even in that setting of an isolation room in the hospital, could, in reality, be having the happiest day that anyone in the world had ever had, or would ever have!

Overflowing with thankfulness to the Lord, love for family, and radiant enthusiasm shared with everyone who came in my room that day, I penned the above sentence with a commitment to seek, pray for, have, and embrace every day to be like that day. Often I fail at having such a day. But, just the remembrance of this sentence and the truth of this sentence awaken my greater senses and sensibilities to the dawn of a spectacular and holy day!

> "Which of you by being anxious can add a single hour to his span of life" (Matt. 6:27)?

> "Therefore do not be anxious about tomorrow, for

tomorrow will be anxious for itself" (Matt. 6:34).

47 The Greatest is Love

Lesson Learned, Opportunity Opened, or Purpose Pursued:

> In Heaven, Love Alone Will Be The Greatest ... Faith and Hope Will No Longer Be Needed Because They Will Be Fulfilled!

"Now these three remain: faith, hope and love. But the greatest of these is love" (1 Corinthians 13:13).

I just noticed (I'm 65 and have been a pastor for 40 years) that of these three (faith, hope, and love), only love is eternal; it, alone among the three, goes on in Heaven forever.

The other two (faith and hope) are gifts in this life to bring us to Heaven where love will be forever.

> There will be no need for faith in Heaven, because "faith is the assurance of things hoped for, the conviction of things not seen" (Hebrews 12:1). In Heaven, we will see "face to face" (1 Cor. 13:12).

> And, there will be no need for hope, because "...hope that is seen is not hope. For who hopes for what he sees" (Rom. 8:24)?

This is love:

> "In this is love, not that we have loved God but that He loved us and sent His Son to be the propitiation for our sins" (1 John 4:10).

48 The Cost

Lesson Learned, Opportunity Opened, or Purpose Pursued:

"You were Ransomed ... Not with Perishable Things Such as Silver or Gold, but with the Precious Blood of Christ..." 1 Peter 1:18-19

A friend, who is also going through lots of medical issues, and I were discussing the high cost of medical treatment.

For example, the experimental drug I am taking, once it hits the market, will be very, very expensive. My first reaction is to look at this as a cost-benefit analysis. I feel a type of guilt or at least patient-angst as I consider the high cost of my treatment.

I am retired, and perhaps my most-productive-to-society days are over, and I could never pay back, in terms of service, the huge cost that has been, and is being, spent on treating my illness. My only justification for receiving the expensive medicine is that perhaps thousands of others may benefit from the scientific knowledge and medical treatments gained by the clinical trial.

But, if the clinical trial only leads to more people using this very, very expensive drug—putting a drain on the whole health system for a questionable benefit (in terms of survival-time and/or improved quality of life), then, again, I feel guilt and angst without any satisfactory justification for such cost in the face of so much other human need.

Then, I think about our Lord's payment for my salvation. Our Lord paid infinitely more than the cost of my experimental drug in order to redeem/save a poor, miserable sinner:

"You know that it was not with perishable things such as silver or gold that you were redeemed from the empty way of life handed down to you from your ancestors, but with the precious blood of Christ" (I Peter 1:18-19).

What's my response to the cost of my salvation? Guilt? Angst? Or, thankfulness, awe, worship, and indebtedness that God would go to that expense/length (sacrifice of His Own and only Son) to save me?

I cannot justify the price our Lord paid for my salvation, but I can thank, praise, serve, and obey Him with the rest of my life, including eternity—a life that He first created and that He now has bought and owns.

I still ask, "Why would God spend so much on me and on each person He saves?" It makes no earthly or human sense. It even causes me to question God's cost-benefit analysis. But, yet, God did pay for our salvation at a humanly unfathomable cost.

Perhaps that is the lesson to be learned in my being treated by this expensive drug—it causes me to understand, just a little bit more, God's GRACE—G-od's R-iches A-t C-hrist's E-xpense.

49 Uncharted Territory - with the Lord

Lesson Learned, Opportunity Opened, or Purpose Pursued:

Fix Our Eyes on Jesus, the Pioneer, as We Face the Future

During yesterday's appointment with my oncologist and my 7th Opdivo infusion during this experimental clinical trial, the doctor reminded me that we are in "uncharted territory" in terms of what could happen month to month.

All of us patients worldwide in this clinical trial (about 300) are marching together in hope for a cure but into uncharted territory.

This reminds me of Hebrews 12:1-2:

> "Since we are surrounded by such a great cloud of witnesses, let us throw off everything that hinders and the sin that so easily entangles. And let us run with perseverance the race marked out for us, fixing our eyes on JESUS, THE PIONEER..."

There is no better Guide to have when entering uncharted territory than Jesus, the Pioneer.

And, isn't every new day uncharted territory for everyone? Therefore, it makes much sense to keep our eyes fixed on Jesus and walk close to Him!

50 An Exchanged Life—Despair for Joy!

Lesson Learned, Opportunity Opened, or Purpose Pursued:

> Live Not Somehow—But Triumphantly!

A purpose-filled life and an "exchanged life" ... "not somehow, but triumphantly!"

A very kind and Christ-like family from Crean Lutheran High School, Irvine, California, (from which I retired nearly two years ago to focus on treatment for the Hodgkin's Lymphoma) has kept in touch with us, prayed for us, and invited us to dinner—again, nearly two years after I stepped away from the school.

How kind! They gave me a book titled, <u>They Found the Secret</u>, a compilation of stories about twenty disciples of Jesus who lived the "exchanged life" (based on Galatians 2:20 and John 10:10)— trading in our human life for life in abundance that is in Jesus. The author, Raymond Edman, had a favorite phrase, "...not somehow, but triumphantly!" I love that.

The kindness this family gave us encourages me to be purposeful (intentional) in living the "exchanged life"—even during this treatment ... "not somehow, but triumphantly" in Christ!

51 OK!

Lesson Learned, Opportunity Opened, or Purpose Pursued:

Come What May, All is OK—with Jesus!

This is a joyful journey, despite three bad days: Aug. 1, 2013, Aug. 6, 2014, May 27, 2015.

- August 1, 2013: My regular doctor, after looking at a chest x-ray taken because I had a cough, told me that I had inoperable cancer spread throughout my lungs.
- August 6, 2014: My oncologist told me that cancer returned after my ABVD chemotherapy which, by the way, usually cures 90% of Hodgkin's Lymphoma patients.
- May 27, 2015: My oncologist told me that despite the stem cell transplant, which usually cures 50% of those who undergo such treatments, the cancer returned.

In spite of these three "bad days," our daily journey is marked by, graced by, and filled with joy from our Lord Jesus, in Whom we have peace that the world cannot give, the certain knowledge of eternal life beyond just this life, and a companion Who is more than sufficient along the way.

Come what may; all is OK—with Jesus.

52 How Powerful is Prayer!

Lesson Learned, Opportunity
Opened, or Purpose Pursued:

Lord, Teach Us To Pray!

How precious is the gift of prayer! Please take a moment to read Charles Spurgeon's comments on prayer from his collection of morning devotions.

> The act of prayer teaches us our unworthiness, which is a very salutary lesson for such proud beings as we are.

> If God gave us favours without constraining us to pray for them we should never know how poor we are, but a true prayer is an inventory of wants, a catalogue of necessities, a revelation of hidden poverty. While it is an application to divine wealth, it is a confession of human emptiness.

> The most healthy state of a Christian is to be always empty in self and constantly depending upon the Lord for supplies; to be always poor in self and rich in Jesus; weak as water personally, but mighty through God to do great exploits; and hence the use of prayer, because, while it adores God, it lays the creature where it should be, in the very dust.

> Prayer is in itself, apart from the answer which it brings, a great benefit to the Christian. As the runner gains strength for the race by daily exercise, so for the great race of life we acquire energy by the hallowed labour of prayer.

> Prayer plumes the wings of God's young eaglets, that they may learn to mount above the clouds.

> Prayer girds the loins of God's warriors, and sends

them forth to combat with their sinews braced and their muscles firm. An earnest pleader cometh out of his closet, even as the sun ariseth from the chambers of the east, rejoicing like a strong man to run his race.

Prayer is that uplifted hand of Moses which routs the Amalekites more than the sword of Joshua; it is the arrow shot from the chamber of the prophet foreboding defeat to the Syrians.

Prayer girds human weakness with divine strength, turns human folly into heavenly wisdom, and gives to troubled mortals the peace of God.

We know not what prayer cannot do! We thank thee, great God, for the mercy-seat, a choice proof of thy marvellous lovingkindness. Help us to use it aright throughout this day!

Charles Spurgeon, October 11 morn.

Prayer:
- Teaches us our unworthiness
- Reminds us of our poverty without Jesus
- Is a confession of our emptiness without Him
- Is a key to divine power
- Points us to the mightiest strength and resource
- "Plumes the wings of God's eaglets"
- Strengthens us for the race, gives peace that the world doesn't know
- And reminds us that we "know not what prayer cannot do."

Lord, "teach us to pray" (Luke 11:1).

53 Beauty Testifies to the Lord!

Lesson Learned, Opportunity Opened, or Purpose Pursued:

The Heavens—and ALL Creation—Declare the Glory of the God!

We went away for a short trip to Sedona, Arizona—where Cindy and I went for our honeymoon over forty years ago. What beauty! The red rock formations are colorful and glorious.

Beauty testifies to the Lord—His goodness, His care and love for His creation (us!) that He would create a world so beautiful for us.

Nature is often called "God's First Book." Psalm 19:1-2 says:

"The heavens declare the glory of God; the skies proclaim the work of his hands. Day after day they pour forth speech; night after night they reveal knowledge."

This "first book" of nature reveals His beauty and goodness and draws us to Him.

His "second" book, the Bible, reveals His Will, His character, His Son Jesus Christ, and our salvation. This sequel, the Bible, is even better than His first book because it is so personal in the revelation of God's character and His Son, Jesus.

In the midst of medical treatment, His revelation, through both of His "books" (nature and the Bible), reminds me that He is a good, loving, and all-powerful Creator, Savior—and even Great Physician.

If He can create the beauty of these red rocks—for us to enjoy—how good and powerful is He over even my illness and life.

54 Waking Up From a Bad Dream— Only to Remember I Have Cancer!

Lesson Learned, Opportunity Opened, or Purpose Pursued:

Which is the True Nightmare—Bad Dreams, When We Wake Up With the Realization We Have Cancer, or Living Without Christ?

I find it almost humorous to often wake up from a nightmare only to realize that I am in a clinical trial for cancer treatment!

Let me explain.

A common theme of many of my dreams (including last night's dream) has been being unprepared (standing in front of a congregation and for some reason not being prepared to give a message or sermon, or finding myself presiding at a wedding and not having the necessary legal documents or not having rehearsed with the couple for what is to come, etc.).

Then, I wake up and find myself—MOMENTARILY—relieved that I am no longer in that stressful situation. But, just as quickly I then remember that I am in a clinical trial for cancer treatment, having failed both chemotherapy and a stem cell transplant.

Bummer!

Chills suddenly run down my spine. Then, I remember that I am in the Lord's hands, and I remember the "Serenity Prayer":

> "God grant me the serenity to accept the things I cannot change, the courage to change the things I can change, and the wisdom to know the difference."

- We have accepted the fact that I have cancer—and have been diagnosed with cancer four times. I cannot change that, so I accept this reality and settle with serenity into this "new normal."

- We have changed what we can change—getting multiple opinions and selecting the best medical treatment, doctors, and medical center that we could. That took not just courage, but lots of time, research, prayer, and ultimately trust in our Lord as we prayerfully sought His guidance in this matter.

- We now daily strive to keep these two tracks from meddling with each other: accepting things we cannot change versus changing things we can change.

The result of this is no longer waking up to a living nightmare, but rather waking up each morning to an exciting and joyous life lived in the peace and presence of Jesus. The real nightmare would be if there were no Jesus Christ.

55 Those who love Jesus

Lesson Learned, Opportunity Opened, or Purpose Pursued:

Grace, Wonders, and Goodness Come to All Who Love Jesus!

A discovery in reading Scripture this morning revealed some promises for "those who love Him [Jesus]." Please read over the following example verses that describe the blessings given to those who love Jesus.

- "Since ancient times no one has heard, no ear has perceived, no eye has seen any God besides you, who acts on behalf of **those who love Him**" (Isaiah 64:4).
- "We know that in all things God works for the good of **those who love Him**, who have been called according to His purpose" (Rom. 8:28).
- "What no eye has seen, nor ear heard, nor the heart of man imagined, what God has prepared for **those who love Him"** (1 Cor. 2:9).
- "Grace to all **who love our Lord Jesus Christ** with an undying love" (Eph. 6:24). That love will never die—and neither will we.

What's our role and job in all this? Love Jesus. That means that our one primary responsibility, both collectively and individually, is to simply love Jesus. Your neighbor, your spouse, your parent, your pastor, or your spiritual counselor cannot love Jesus for you.

Each of us has one ultimate purpose, role, job, and Calling: love Jesus.

What is our Lord's promised part and role for those who love Him?

- **He acts on behalf** of those who love Him,

- In all things, **He works for the good** of those who love Him,
- **He prepares wonders** God for those who love Him,
- **He gives grace** for those who love our Lord Jesus Christ.

56 Wake Up!

Lesson Learned, Opportunity Opened, or Purpose Pursued:

> Be Fully Alive—More Than Just Having a Beating Heart!

While on this morning's bike ride, I realized that for the past 27 months, 2.25 years, I have not been sick—other than of course the cancer/Hodgkin's Lymphoma.

No flu, no colds, no runny noses.

How ironic; I have a cancer that has not responded to two traditional treatments (chemotherapy and a stem cell transplant), and yet I have "not been sick" for over two years.

What a parable of life! How many of us think we are healthy (no colds, no flu, etc.), and yet we do not realize the terminal and eternal-sin-sick peril that afflicts all of us outside of Christ?

This reminds me of Revelation 3:1-2:

> "...you have a reputation of being alive, but you are dead. Wake up!"

May we all "wake up" to the fact that only "in Christ" are we alive and well, whether physically healthy or gravely sick, whether heretofore aware or unaware of our true eternal relationship in Christ.

57 Knowing the Difference

Lesson Learned, Opportunity
Opened, or Purpose Pursued:

Dear Lord, Please Grant Me Both Serenity and Courage.

How important it is to seek and to keep the truth spoken in the famous "Serenity Prayer" in mind:

> "God grant me the serenity to accept the things I cannot change, the courage to change the things I can change, and the wisdom to know the difference."

In the clinical trial in which I am enrolled, I cannot change the ultimate outcome.

BUT, that does not relegate me to a fatalistic acceptance of a medical outcome influenced by no outside force.

The "acceptance of things I cannot change" gloriously includes God's sovereign grace—which rules over me, over the world, and even over cancer.

The "courage to change the things I can change" includes everything over which I have control—my daily attitude, my daily prayers, the food I eat, the sleep I get, the exercise I do, the compliance to my doctor's guidance that he gives.

Dear Lord, please grant me both serenity and courage.

58 In Christ in this World versus Safely Home in Heaven

Lesson Learned, Opportunity Opened, or Purpose Pursued:

> One of the Holiest Moments of a Christian's Life is to Acknowledge, at a Christian's Passing, "Another One Safely Home!"

My wife's mother died this past week.

A few years ago, after serving as a parish pastor for thirty years, I made a list of the "Top 10 Joys of Parish Ministry."

In that list was the thought and accompanying peaceful feeling I always had when walking away from a graveside service of a believer as I would always say, as a prayer and a statement of praise to the Lord,

"Another one safely home."

This side of Heaven, we live "in Christ."

On the other side of death, we live at "home" with Christ (John 14:1-6).

On both sides of death, our protection, our joy, and our safety are all found "in Christ."

I often sign emails and letters with the closing, "In Christ (...the best, safest, and most joyful place to be!), Pastor Bill."

Indeed, "in Christ" is the best place to be on both sides of earthly death.

But, how much safer will we all be when we are eternally home with, in, and through Christ!

59 An Advantaged State

Lesson Learned, Opportunity
Opened, or Purpose Pursued:

> There is a Blessedness and an Advantage in Being Aware of Our Human Mortality through Treatment and Trials

Last night, Cindy and I attended an annual Crean Lutheran High School Christmas Concert.

As we listened to the beautiful, traditional carols such as:

- "Of the Father's Love Begotten"
- "Angels from the Realms of Glory"
- "Away in a Manger"
- "O Come, O Come Emmanuel" and
- "O Come, All Ye Faithful"

I had a revelation:

- If we sing of and believe in the subject content of these beautiful hymns and carols
- If indeed Jesus is our Savior and that He came to redeem us from a life of suffering and sin through His death on the Cross and resurrection, and,
- If our final joy is indeed "in Christ"—with Him forever in the "realms of glory",

then, without sounding morbid, I, in my condition of being in a clinical trial for recurrent cancer, am in an advantaged state of perhaps being closer to that "realm of glory."

If what we sing about, read about, pray for, and trust in is eternal life and presence with Jesus, then my condition—or any earthly suffering or illness—is not so bad after all.

As a matter of fact, the glorious beauty of worship experienced in that Christmas concert last night was just a poor foretaste, BUT a REAL foretaste, of a reality that is so glorious and wonderful that no artist or musician on earth could do it justice.

"Amen. Come, Lord Jesus" (Rev. 22:20).

60 Already and Yet to Come!

Lesson Learned, Opportunity Opened, or Purpose Pursued:

The Christian Life is Based on So Much that Jesus Already Did, But it Also Overflows with Joyous Anticipation Into What is Yet to Come!

Christians live both fulfilled here and now and in anticipation of even greater fulfillment!

In this year's Advent devotions ("The Dawning of Indestructible Joy" by John Piper), the fulfillment of Biblical prophecy was discussed in a devotion dated December 13. Too many Christians practice an "either/or" Christianity. Either they focus on what blessings we have been given already and forget the glories yet to come; or, they do not appreciate or appropriate the blessings given to us in this life and only focus on the coming Kingdom of Heaven. Jesus has given us blessings beyond imagining both in the here and now as well as in the eternal life to come! How rich we are!

This side of Heaven is already FULL of fulfilled prophecies and promises:

- The incarnation
- The crucifixion
- The atonement
- Complete propitiation
- The resurrection
- The ascension
- Christ's heavenly reign
- Intercession by Jesus and the Holy Spirit
- The outpouring of the Holy Spirit

- The far-reaching global missions
- The ingathering of the nations
- The Church as the Body of Christ
- The witness of the New Testament Scriptures
- Personal prayer in Jesus' name
- Joy unspeakable
- And absolute certainty of our future in Heaven has been purchased and is secure!

What joy and fulfillment is already ours! What peace this gives even during this time of frail flesh and uncertain future.

And yet, there is still so much more to come! We look forward to and anticipate with eager joy:

- The second coming
- The resurrection of the dead
- New and glorious bodies
- The end of sinning
- Living in the glory of the presence of our Lord
- Judgment on all unbelief
- Rewards
- Entrance into the Master's joy
- New heavens and new earth
- Jesus present among his people face-to-face
- No more misery, and
- Pleasures forevermore

We are double-blessed—already living in so many fulfilled promises —and so many more yet to come!

61 For His Glory

Lesson Learned, Opportunity Opened, or Purpose Pursued:

Blessings, Answers to Prayers, and Favor from the Lord ALWAYS Have One Purpose or End in Mind: to Enable the Recipient/Believer to Glorify and Praise the Lord!

Last evening's Advent devotion, from "The Dawning of Indestructible Joy" by John Piper, made another obvious but seldom acknowledged observation:

Blessings, answers to prayers, and favor from the Lord ALWAYS have one purpose or end in mind: to enable the recipient of salvation/the believer to glorify and praise the Lord.

- What is forgiveness other than removing a hindrance that keeps the believer from the glorious presence of the Lord?
- What is a blessing if not an opportunity to draw nearer to Christ?
- What is the gift of sanctification if not the purifying of our praises?
- What is physical healing if not the gift of more opportunity to bring glory to Jesus?

We were created "for His glory" (Isaiah 43:7), so it is proper that the more like our original intent we become through Christ's grace, the purer our praises and purposes become.

Let us together, and always, praise the Lord!

62 Pray to be Different!

Lesson Learned, Opportunity Opened, or Purpose Pursued:

The Illness May Not Be Different, But the Patient Is!

Today, in a book containing several biographies about faithful Christians, I read about Dwight Moody.

After the Lord had worked in Dwight Moody a deepened faith, Moody made the following comment about the impact this deepened faith had in his life,

"The sermon was not different, but the servant was."

A theme from his biography was that he found it incredulous that so many Christians pray for forgiveness and salvation—and nothing more.

Should we not seek and pray for sanctification and holiness with the same urgency and fervency as we seek and pray for forgiveness and salvation?

Applying this to my situation, the following statements can be made:

- The illness may or may not be different in the future, but I pray that the patient and the disciple (I) will be different! That difference is the deepest healing from the Lord.
- Should we not seek and pray for a healed spirit and soul with the same urgency and fervency as we seek and pray for physical healing?

63 Heaven and Christ

Lesson Learned, Opportunity
Opened, or Purpose Pursued:

> "O Lord, Heaven Without Thee Would be Hell!"
> -Samuel Rutherford

In Charles Spurgeon's morning devotion for January 17, based on Revelation 14:1, Spurgeon quoted this famous assertion made by Samuel Rutherford, back in the 17th century:

> "Heaven and Christ are the same thing; to be with Christ is to be in heaven, and to be in heaven is to be with Christ. O my Lord Jesus Christ, if I could be in heaven without Thee, it would be a hell; and if I could be in hell, and have Thee still, it would be a heaven to me, for Thou art all the heaven I want."

Would that we all, and at all times, could have that singleness of vision and passion!

64 Pray and Never Give Up!

Lesson Learned, Opportunity Opened, or Purpose Pursued:

> Always Pray and Never Give Up!

"Jesus told His disciples ... that they should always pray and not give up" (Luke 18:1).

Great advice from Jesus!

- Always pray.
- Never give up.

Oh, how our lives would be better if only we followed these few words of instruction—which are also an invitation to grace.

If we pray always, we'll understand, have, and radiate the peace of Christ which passes all human understanding, and we'll be both a sign and presence of Jesus and His coming/already here Kingdom!

If we never give up, we'll discover for ourselves and witness to others that our Lord Jesus Christ provides strength sufficient for each moment, each suffering, and each treatment. If we never give up, we will be that consistent and persistent witness to others who are undergoing similar suffering to also follow these words of instruction and invitation to His grace:

- Always pray. Never give up.

65 That Man

Lesson Learned, Opportunity
Opened, or Purpose Pursued:

> We are Here to Talk About a Man— That Man is Jesus
> -Paul Scalia

Being in a clinical trial, I am attentive to memorial services.

Today, February 20, 2016, was the funeral mass for Supreme Court Justice Antonin Scalia.

Scalia was a very faithful Christian and an impressive, intelligent, respected and well-liked Supreme Court justice. Even his political opponents respected and liked him.

Scalia's funeral mass was given by one of his nine children, a Roman Catholic priest named Paul. What a powerful witness and message he gave! Here is a link to the full eulogy, which notes that it was because of "one man" that they were gathered together: https://www.firstthings.com/web-exclusives/2016/02/funeral-homily-for-justice-antonin-scalia

What a wonderful eulogy. What a wonderful proclamation of Jesus Christ. What a wonderful legacy of a disciple of Christ.

At my memorial service, I want the main topic of it, both of the service and the message, to be "about that man—Jesus Christ." To that end, I've mentioned this before and I state it again: St. Anselm's quote read at my memorial service. (See prior chapter titled, "Your Final Answer.")

66 Free to Serve!

Lesson Learned, Opportunity Opened, or Purpose Pursued:

Living "On The Precipice" Can Be Exciting and Holy!

Being 75% of a year (week 39) into this clinical trial, and settling into a realization that, by God's grace, my immediate health and life may not be as at-risk as they were one year ago, I feel a freeing excitement about the future in two ways:

- First, there is a combined sense of exhilaration and peace that "living on the precipice" gives. One the one hand, the prospect of extended life and health is exciting; on the other hand, the alternative is not bad. As a matter of fact, since Scripture is true, departing this life is better. So excitement awaits me either way. This "living on the precipice" enhances life in ways that may not be experienced without this awareness.

- Second, being retired gives me a sense of having completed the phase of "preparation" in my life. Just like finishing college or finishing a residency, I have now been prepared and set free to be attentive to opportunities to serve the Lord and others. I no longer "have to work" or "make a living." Our retirement savings and income allow me to be self-funded in offering myself and/or my labors in pursuit of what I sense the Lord's Call to me to be. I can now respond immediately and in creative ways—consulting, serving, supporting —to any ministry need or prompt of Jesus that may come my way.

How exciting and holy is all of life? How blessed are we all!

67 Running With Focus

Lesson Learned, Opportunity Opened, or Purpose Pursued:

Keep Eyes Fixed On Jesus and Run With Perseverance -- and With His Energy!

Yesterday, in church, one of the lessons read during worship was from Philippians 3:

> "I press on to take hold of that for which Christ Jesus took hold of me. Brothers and sisters, I do not consider myself yet to have taken hold of it. But one thing I do: Forgetting what is behind and straining toward what is ahead, I press on toward the goal to win the prize for which God has called me heavenward in Christ Jesus" (Philippians 3:12-14).

I love that passage. It reminds me of a race—running and keeping our eyes and thoughts on the goal of being with Jesus! Throughout this journey of cancer and its treatment, I have experienced many of the emotions that long distance runners know well:

- I felt exhaustion!
- I "hit the wall"—a few times!
- I suffered through blisters—not on my feet but from my lips and mouth all the through my entire gastrointestinal tract!
- I didn't know if I could finish the race!

Yet, the Lord has refreshed me and strengthened me along the way. His grace, like refreshing and still waters, restored my soul. He never left me and never forsook me! And, He continues to faithfully provide this daily support!

This passage from Philippians reminds me of three other passages that also compare the life of faith with the experience of running a race with distractions and sufferings all around. These verses remind us to keep our eyes fixed on Jesus, Whose energy (not ours, but His) keeps us going all the way to Heaven.

- "Therefore, since we are surrounded by such a great cloud of witnesses, let us throw off everything that hinders and the sin that so easily entangles. And let us run with perseverance the race marked out for us, fixing our eyes on Jesus..." (Heb. 12:1-2).

- "To this end (the GOAL of being with Jesus) I strenuously contend with all the energy Christ so powerfully works in me" (Col. 1:29).

- "I consider my life worth nothing to me; my only aim is to finish the race and complete the task the Lord Jesus has given me—the task of testifying to the good news of God's grace" (Acts 20:24).

Let us together run this race and keep our eyes fixed on Jesus!

68 Not He, But You

Lesson Learned, Opportunity Opened, or Purpose Pursued:

> The 23rd Psalm's Reminder That our Lord is Closer than 3rd Person!

Here's a great thought about prayer—using the 23rd Psalm. Note that verses 1-3 all deal with the Lord in the third person ("He").

Then, note that at the end of verse 4, when talking about the valley of the shadow of death, the pronoun case changes to 2nd person ("You").

> "The Lord is my shepherd, I shall not want. 2 <u>He</u> makes me lie down in green pastures; <u>He</u> leads me beside quiet waters. 3 <u>He</u> restores my soul; <u>He</u> guides me in the paths of righteousness for His name's sake. 4 Even though I walk through the valley of the shadow of death, I fear no evil, for <u>You are with me</u>; <u>Your rod and Your staff, they comfort me.</u> 5 <u>You prepare</u> a table before me in the presence of my enemies; <u>You have anointed</u> my head with oil; My cup overflows. 6 Surely goodness and lovingkindness will follow me all the days of my life, And I will dwell in the house of the Lord forever."

I love that! When life really gets tough, we cannot just talk about some 3rd person's help; we need to talk personally to our Lord and Savior, saying, "YOU COMFORT, YOU PREPARE, YOU ANOINT, YOU ARE WITH ME!

Our Lord wants—and provides—a 1st and 2nd person, intimate relationship with us. A distant, 3rd person relationship does not comfort—especially when facing valleys with dark shadows.

Thank YOU, Jesus.

69 Enough is Enough!

Lesson Learned, Opportunity Opened, or Purpose Pursued:

Jesus is Enough, and Jesus Will Determine When it is Enough!

Today is my 66th birthday.

Here are a couple of thoughts:

- My mother died from cancer at age 46. Every birthday, I remember that my mother—a very good and faithful lady—died much younger than I currently am. I realize how every year is a gift.

- This morning's Charles Spurgeon devotion, for May 2, was based on John 17:15:

    "I pray not that thou shouldst take them out of the world, but that You keep them from the evil one. They are not of the world, just as I am not of the world."

- This verse assures me that Jesus' grace is enough strength for me "in this world."

The last lines of Spurgeon's devotion are:

    "...to be with Christ is far better, but the wish to escape from trouble is a selfish one. Rather let your care and wish be to glorify God by your life here as long as He pleases, even though it be in the midst of toil, and conflict, and suffering, and leave Him to say when 'it is enough.'"

The Lord has already allowed me to live twenty years longer than did my mother. On the one hand, that is more than enough—more than I could expect. But, the Lord has not yet said, "it is enough"—so I will keep serving, praising, and proclaiming until He does!

Indeed, God's grace is always "enough"—on earth or in Heaven. Thank You, Lord, for another year.

70 Words: "Direct" versus "Guide"

Lesson Learned, Opportunity
Opened, or Purpose Pursued:

I Need our Lord's Direction More Than I Need His Guidance!

My favorite picture (which to this day prominently hangs above our fireplace) is Sallman's "Christ our Pilot." It is a beautiful image of a young man at the helm of a ship in the midst of a wild storm. Waves can be seen crashing into the boat, yet there is a patch of blue in the storm-cloud sky, promising hope. The young man is resolutely holding the ship's wheel. Behind him is Jesus with His left hand on the young man's shoulder and with His right hand piloting the way. I love this picture.

But, recently, I have intentionally been praying for our Lord's direction rather than guidance—thinking about this picture.

- Definition: "Guide: show or indicate the way to (someone)."
- Definition: "Direct: control the operations of; manage or govern."

I need Jesus' "direction"—to control, manage, govern, and pilot my life. I fear how I may respond to just "guidance"—and how I so easily and quickly could (or would!) reject that "showing" or "indicating."

Lord Jesus, please be my pilot and direct my paths!

"Trust in the Lord with all your heart, and lean not on your own understanding; in all your ways acknowledge Him, and He shall direct your paths" (Proverbs 3:5-6 NKJV).

71 The Word "Deign"

Lesson Learned, Opportunity Opened, or Purpose Pursued:

How Wonderful That Our Lord "Deigns" to Love, Redeem, and Save Us!

I learned a new word by reading Charles Spurgeon's morning devotions. The word is "deign."

Definition: "Deign: do something that one considers to be beneath one's dignity, condescend to give (something)."

Charles Spurgeon often used this word in his writing to describe our Lord's grace shown to us. Spurgeon's evening devotion for March 21 is one example. Here is an excerpt from that devotion:

> "In the spiritual, as in the natural world, man's power is limited on all hands. When the Holy Spirit sheds abroad his delights in the soul, none can disturb; all the cunning and malice of men are ineffectual to stay the genial quickening power of the Comforter. When [the Lord] deigns to visit a church and revive it, the most inveterate enemies cannot resist the good work; they may ridicule it, but they can no more restrain it than they can push back the spring when the Pleiades rule the hour."

"Deign" is a word used to describe our Lord's condescension to meet us, minister to us, strengthen us, die for us, and redeem us.

How wonderful that our Lord "deigns" to love, redeem, and save us.

72 Hezekiah's Added 15 Years

Lesson Learned, Opportunity
Opened, or Purpose Pursued:

> Wholehearted Devotion and Hezekiah's Prayer.

I have to admit that I have thought of Hezekiah, King of Judah, several times during my bouts with cancer.

In both 2 Kings 20 and Isaiah 38, we read accounts of Hezekiah and an illness that threatened his life. Upon hearing news of his mortal illness, Hezekiah immediately turned his face to the wall and prayed to, begged, and implored the Lord. The Lord heard and answered Hezekiah's prayer—adding fifteen years to his life.

> "Then the word of the Lord came to Isaiah: "Go and say to Hezekiah, Thus says the Lord, the God of David your father: I have heard your prayer; I have seen your tears. Behold, I will add fifteen years to your life" (Isaiah 38: 4-5).

Let us be encouraged in this account. The Lord hears the prayers of His children who humble themselves, turn to Him and pour out their hearts to Him.

While our prayers do not dictate the gracious actions and mercy of our Lord, our prayers are received by a very personal and loving God Who invites us, begs us, and implores us to pray to Him! Like Hezekiah, let us immediately turn to the Lord in prayer.

Lessons learned: pray. The Lord is gracious and merciful, and He answers prayer.

73 Lonesome Valley

Lesson Learned, Opportunity
Opened, or Purpose Pursued:

> Even While Walking that Lonesome Valley, "Thou Art With Me"!

Remember the old song, "Lonesome Valley," by Woody Guthrie?

Unless you were born in the mid-20th century or earlier, you probably don't. Nevertheless, consider the words of this song, starting with the first stanza:

> "You gotta walk that lonesome valley, You gotta walk it
> by yourself, Nobody here can walk it for you, You gotta
> walk it by yourself."

I still have vivid memories of singing this song to myself as I would struggle to walk around the block back in 1983 during my first bout with cancer when I was undergoing chemotherapy.

On one particular occasion, I didn't know if I could make it around the block. It was in Phoenix—in the summer. It was hot. Midway around the block, I ran out of strength. I sat on the curb and thought of this song and how this walk was the parable of all of life.

I was alone at that moment—at least alone in terms of fellow human pilgrims. But, then I remembered Psalm 23, especially verse 4, "Even though I walk through the valley of the shadow of death, I will fear no evil, for You are with me."

Since that moment and that walk, this song has actually been a comfort to me and a reminder to me that all people have to walk that "lonesome valley" (LIFE!) ultimately alone, even though they may be surrounded by family, friends, and medical caregivers. But, the precious Gospel message in all this is that while we may be alone in a human sense, we are never alone because our Good Shepherd is with us even when we walk through the "valley of the shadow."

The words of the other stanzas reinforce this message. http://woodyguthrie.org/Lyrics/Lonesome_Valley.htm

Strangely, I find comfort in this—knowing that Jesus will never, ever leave or forsake me. What a wonderful ever-present Savior!

74 Assurance Verses

Lesson Learned, Opportunity Opened, or Purpose Pursued:

Bible Promises You Can Take to the Grave—and then to Heaven!

I've mentioned in previous chapters that I love "memory verses." Even more than "memory verses," I love what I call "assurance verses." As a pastor, many times I have called and recited one or more of these "assurance verses" to patients and family members during holy and critical times of life-threatening circumstances.

"Assurance verses" are promises from God's Word that His grace in Christ is sufficient for salvation and the gift of Heaven for the believer.

- Jesus said, "Truly, truly, I say to you, whoever hears My word and believes Him Who sent Me has eternal life. He does not come into judgment, but has passed from death to life" (John 5:24).
- "If you confess with your mouth that Jesus is Lord and believe in your heart that God raised Him from the dead, you will be saved" (Rom. 10:9).
- "To all who did receive [Jesus], who believed in His name, He gave the right to become children of God, who were born, not of blood nor of the will of the flesh nor of the will of man, but of God" (John 1:12-13).
- "Whoever comes to Me I will never cast out...everyone who looks on the Son and believes in Him should have eternal life, and I will raise him up on the last day" (John 6:37 & 40).

What blessed assurance these verses give during times of life-threatening illnesses or circumstances! I pray that these verses also

give you full assurance of salvation and eternal life through Jesus
Christ.

75 A Gift and a Privilege!

Lesson Learned, Opportunity
Opened, or Purpose Pursued:

> To be Able to Exercise—Riding a Bike in the Lord's Beautiful Outdoors—is a Gift and a Privilege!

Often, when something is taken away or threatened to be taken away, it becomes more cherished.

Exercise, for me, is one of those activities! During my treatment, regular exercise has been a gift and a privilege!

Exercise has always been important to me. As a matter of fact, I wrestled in junior high, high school, and college, and after that, as an "old timer," with local high school and college wrestling teams up until the year of diagnosis of Hodgkin's Lymphoma. (Yes, that means I was wrestling when I was way "over the hill"!)

By God's grace, I am still able to exercise during treatment, and I do so about five days every week.

Every time—EVERY TIME—during my exercise (either a bike ride or elliptical), I exclaim—sometimes out loud, "What a gift and a privilege!"

There have been times during my treatment when I was not able to exercise—or just plain physically couldn't exercise. To be able to exercise, to sweat, to be outdoors (when biking), to be fully alive and enjoying life is a precious gift and privilege.

May I never look at exercise—or any other "normal" activity, even including household chores or yard work—as a burden, but always as a gift and privilege from the Lord.

"This [and every opportunity in this day!] is the day [and gift] that the Lord has made; let us rejoice and be glad in it" (Psalm 118:24)!

76 Tethered and Thankful

Lesson Learned, Opportunity
Opened, or Purpose Pursued:

> Even "Bad News" Can Be a Blessing As It Tethers Us
> Closer to Christ!

Today I received the 25th infusion of Opdivo—approaching one year in this clinical trial.

I also received the radiology report for the scan I had yesterday. The report indicated a new nodule in my lower right lung and a nodule in my upper chest. The doctor said that both are too small to worry about at this point and that we will just be aware of and watch these in our future appointments.

This certainly was not "bad news" compared to other genuinely "bad news" reports I have had in the past. Nevertheless, news like this keeps one tethered in prayer to the Lord and attentive to the blessings of each day.

After the appointment, I find that I am leaning a little more into the Lord and that I am more sensitive to the blessings of today.

I guess it was a good day after all—tethered and thankful to Christ!

77 Not Just Now, But Always

Lesson Learned, Opportunity Opened, or Purpose Pursued:

Not Just Now. I Desperately Need the Lord and His Grace ALWAYS.

In today's Charles Spurgeon's morning devotion (May 25), we are reminded that there is never a moment when we are not in need of our Lord's presence, redeeming, guiding, and protecting.

A couple of sentences from Spurgeon's devotion emphasize this truth:

- "There is no moment of our life, however holy, in which we can do without his constant upholding."
- "Forsake me not, for my path is dangerous, and full of snares, and I cannot do without thy guidance."

Let me never forget that my needs for our Lord's salvation and moment-by-moment safe-keeping, now so well known to me during this cancer treatment, were just as great before cancer and will be just as great after cancer if I am cured.

"Forsake me not, O Lord" (Psalm 38:21) —anytime!

78 God's Will

Lesson Learned, Opportunity Opened, or Purpose Pursued:

> God's Will Wills the Good!

My mother died of cancer when she was forty-six years old and I was twenty-four years old. Her death impacted my life in many ways. In the days following her passing, a friend of our family sent us a card in which was printed the following challenging, inspiring, and compelling perspectives:

> "It is God's Will," he meekly said, and bowed a weak submissive head.
>
> Folding his hands with passive grace, he yielded his place in life's race.
>
> "There is no more that I can do; my life has ended, I am through!"
>
> His head hanging toward the setting sun, vanquished he said, "God's Will be done."
>
> His brother said, "It is God's Will that I continue useful still.
>
> Perhaps I cannot work or live the same, but there is still much in life to gain!
>
> God has not willed this pain of mine; these handicaps are not divine.
>
> God wills the good! Life is not always understood! I believe that God wills that I should keep on serving till I die."
>
> His face turned toward the rising sun, with eager zeal,

he said, "God's Will be done!"

What a difference in perspective these two paths or points of view offer us!

Dear fellow cancer patient or caregiver: Let us together encourage each other to choose the latter perspective! Our Lord does indeed desire us to continue useful still! Our lives are surely not the same as they once were, but there is still much good for us to do in this life! These illnesses and pains are not from the Lord; they are the result of a fallen creation, the complexity and course of which we simply cannot understand. Meanwhile, the Lord has great purposes for us ... and great graces and mercies and blessings for us! Let us together boldly, loudly, enthusiastically, and daily say, in word and deed, "God's Will be done in and through my life!"

79 Read!

Lesson Learned, Opportunity Opened, or Purpose Pursued:

> Christian Books Can Help You ...Not Escape ...But Be Set Free!

Ecclesiastes 12:12 tells us that even three thousand years ago... "of making many books there is no end...." And, if that was three thousand years ago, how much more so now with the availability of thousands of new books each month and now with e-books making them so much more convenient!

Cancer treatment often gives the patient and the caregiver more time. It seems "waiting" is part and parcel of enduring illness and treatment.

In acknowledgment of this truth, I am sharing with you—and commending to you—some books which have ministered to me over the past three years when I have been enduring treatment. I've read many more, but these "Top Ten" have been insightful, helpful, and encouraging to me—and, I hope, they may be equally so to you.

1. *Surprised by Suffering*, R.C. Sproul
2. *Finishing our Course with Joy*, J.I. Packer
3. *Grace*, Max Lucado
4. *The Joy of the Gospel*, Pope Francis
5. *The Reason for My Hope*, Billy Graham
6. *The Question that Never Goes Away*, Philip Yancey
7. *Jesus, the Only Way to God*, John Piper
8. *They Found the Secret*, V. Raymond Edman
9. *The Pursuit of God*, A. W. Tozer
10. *The Name of God is Mercy*, Pope Francis

80 Something Greater!

Lesson Learned, Opportunity Opened, or Purpose Pursued:

> What a Privilege to be a Part of Something Greater -- Both Here on Earth and in Heaven Forever!

One could lament being enrolled in a clinical trial. Being in a clinical trial usually means that prior treatment has failed and that the disease is progressing.

However, what a joy it is to be a part of a team (research scientists, lab assistants, doctors, nurses, pharmaceutical companies, investors, etc.) working on cures for dreaded diseases like cancer.

As a patient enrolled in a clinical trial, I have been given an important role to fill in a search for curing cancer. This adds joy, anticipation, purpose, and peace to this journey.

Even more joyous is the certainty of being enrolled in the Book of Life in Heaven!

> "Rejoice that your names are written in heaven" (Luke 10:20).

This, too, is part of a cure—an eternal cure that will erase all sickness, tears, and dying.

> "He will wipe away every tear from their eyes, and death shall be no more, neither shall there be mourning, nor crying, nor pain anymore, for the former things have passed away" (Revelation 21:4).

Enrolled in the clinical trial and on the roster of our Lord's Book of Life! What a joy to be on these two teams!

81 Medicine of Immortality

Lesson Learned, Opportunity
Opened, or Purpose Pursued:

Where the Body and Blood of our Lord Jesus Christ are,
May There be Found no Iniquity or illness Within Me.

The above words are those a kind Christian physician once
gave to me to guide my prayers as I prepare to receive the Lord's
Supper during worship.

Ever since this doctor of both body and soul spoke these words
to me, I have uttered variations of this prayer every time I prepare
to receive the Sacrament.

Over the course of my treatment, this short prayer has expanded
to something similar to the following paraphrase whenever I
receive the Sacrament of Holy Communion:

> "Dear Lord, as I receive Your Body and Blood, Your
> Holy Word and Sacrificial atonement, Your power
> and Your Holy Spirit, Your Resurrection and gift of
> regeneration, and You as Lord and Savior, may there
> be found no iniquity, no sin, no cancer, no illness,
> no anything that diminishes Your holiness within or
> through me. Amen."

82 Holy Words: "Even if ... Yet..."

Lesson Learned, Opportunity Opened, or Purpose Pursued:

> "Even if He Does Not..." "Yet Will I Rejoice in the Lord..."

There are many heroes and saints in Christian history. I would like to highlight four Biblical heroes who inspire me: Shadrach, Meshach, and Abednego—three deportees from Jerusalem to Babylon—and the prophet Habakkuk.

As you read in context the following paragraphs and underlined expressions of deep, deep trust and faith uttered by these four heroes, please consider situations in your life in which you are suffering or in which you have great need and for which you have cried out to the Lord for rescue. Are you willing, even if Jesus does not come to your rescue, to say, "Even if He does not...yet will I rejoice in the Lord"?

> "Nebuchadnezzar said to [Shadrach, Meshach, and Abednego], "If you are ready when you hear the sound of the horn, pipe, lyre, trigon, harp, bagpipe, and every kind of music, to fall down and worship the image that I have made, well and good. But if you do not worship, you shall immediately be cast into a burning fiery furnace." Shadrach, Meshach, and Abednego answered and said to the king, "O Nebuchadnezzar, we have no need to answer you in this matter. If this be so, our God whom we serve is able to deliver us from the burning fiery furnace, and He will deliver us out of your hand, O king. But <u>even if He does not</u>, be it known to you, O king, that we will not serve your gods or worship the golden image that you have set up" (Daniel 3:13-18, excerpts).

"Though the fig tree should not blossom, nor fruit be on the vines, the produce of the olive fail and the fields yield no food, the flock be cut off from the fold and there be no herd in the stalls, <u>yet</u> I will rejoice in the Lord; I will take joy in the God of my salvation" (Habakkuk 3:17-18).

Dear Lord Jesus, help us to trust in You and to have deep faith in You "even if" You, in Your omniscience and grace, do not respond to our cries for help in ways that we desire. May we "yet" rejoice in, praise, and trust in You. Amen.

83 The Cross

Lesson Learned, Opportunity Opened, or Purpose Pursued:

O Lord, Let My Life Point to You!

While on an Alaska trip that we squeezed between clinical trial treatments, we stopped to visit a historical site, St. Nicholas Russian Orthodox Church, an early original church building dating back to 1893, in Juneau.

As we stepped into the small, yet well-kept 100+-year-old church, we were greeting by a Russian Orthodox deacon in full vestments. He was there to welcome visitors, give a history of St. Nicholas Russian Orthodox Church, and to answer questions. He did all this graciously and with great and interesting detail.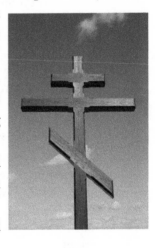

We learned an interesting and meaningful fact about the symbolism of the Russian Orthodox Cross.

The cross has three horizontal crossbeams:

- The top one represents the plate which in the older Greek tradition is inscribed with a phrase based on John's Gospel "The King of Glory." In older Christian history and still in non-Orthodox tradition, this top "plate" was frequently depicted with the letters INRI, referencing the first letters of the main words of "Jesus of Nazareth, King of the Jews" (John 19:19).

- The middle cross beam is the traditional horizontal piece of the cross onto which the arms of Jesus were fastened by nails or spikes.
- In the Russian Orthodox tradition, there is a third crossbeam, which is slanted.
  - The side to Christ's right is tilted higher. This is because this footrest slants upward toward the penitent thief traditionally known as St. Dismas, who was crucified on Jesus' right. The upward slant is also traditionally interpreted as pointing toward Heaven.
  - The left side of the lower crossbeam is slanted downward toward the impenitent thief, traditionally known as Gestas. The downward slant is also traditionally interpreted as pointing toward hell.

One of the Orthodox Church's prayers appointed for Friday prayers further interprets the cross' symbolism:

> "In the midst, between two thieves, was Your Cross found as the balance-beam of righteousness; For while one was led down to hell by the burden of his blaspheming, the other was lightened of his sins unto the knowledge of things divine, O Christ God glory to You."

My prayer, paraphrased from a prayer of an anonymous Christian saint:

Dear Lord Jesus, my most ardent desire is not for position given to David, nor favor given to Nehemiah, nor healing given to the paralytic, nor title given to Peter; but that forgiveness You granted to the thief on the Cross—that is my greatest desire. Amen.

84 Bequeathed to Us

Lesson Learned, Opportunity Opened, or Purpose Pursued:

> The Greatest Riches and Treasures of J.P. Morgan are Ours as Well!

Yesterday, I read the following in a devotional book. J.P. Morgan, the multi-millionaire, who died in 1913, had a will that contained 10,000 words, including instructions for many transactions and tasks upon his death.

Among the 10,000 words, the following was the most important part of his will:

> "I commit my soul into the hands of my Savior, in full confidence that, having redeemed and washed it in His most precious blood, He will present it faultless before my Heavenly Father, and I entreat my children to maintain and defend, at all hazard and at any cost of personal sacrifice, the blessed doctrine of the complete atonement for sin through the blood of Jesus Christ, once offered, and through that alone."

J. P. Morgan's greatest treasure and true wealth were reflected in this paragraph. That treasure was Jesus Christ. What treasure … what an inheritance … is bequeathed to us!

> "Where your treasure is, there will your heart be also" (Matthew 6:21).

That same treasure and same wealth belong to everyone who knows and loves Jesus Christ—even to you and me! How rich we are in Christ!

85 Cheerful Holiness

Lesson Learned, Opportunity Opened, or Purpose Pursued:

Cheerful Holiness is an Infectious Contagion!

"Cheerful holiness." What a great aspiration. What a great witness. What a great disposition. What an infectious contagion. Charles Spurgeon, in his August 14 Morning Devotion, reflecting on Psalm 92:4, "Thou, Lord, hast made me glad through thy work," overflows with the joy of Christ's completed work of salvation accomplished on the Cross for the believer.

This one gift—forgiveness of sins (atonement)—enables the believer to endure, overcome, and even rejoice in the midst of anything else that may occur in this life. Quoting Martin Luther, the 16th-century reformer, Spurgeon even taunts the many threats that this world throws at us:

> "'Smite, Lord, smite, for my sin is forgiven; if Thou hast but forgiven me, smite as hard as thou wilt;' and in a similar spirit you may say, 'Send sickness, poverty, losses, crosses, persecution, what thou wilt, thou hast forgiven me, and my soul is glad.'"

Toward the end of his devotion, Spurgeon writes, "Holy gladness and holy boldness will make you a good preacher, and all the world will be a pulpit... Cheerful holiness is the most forcible of sermons."

Cheerful holiness is a frame of mind that belongs to, and flows from, God's children.

86 In the Company of Caleb and Joshua

Lesson Learned, Opportunity
Opened, or Purpose Pursued:

> "He (the Lord) will bring us into this land"!
> Numbers 14:8

Numbers 13 contains the account of the Lord's command to Moses to send twelve spies to explore the Promised Land. The twelve were chosen, one from each tribe, and they together, as pioneers, explored the land, returned, and reported what they found.

Ten of the twelve were fearful about entering the land:

> "'We can't attack those people! They're too strong for us!' So they began to spread lies among the Israelites about the land they had explored. They said, 'The land we explored is one that devours those who live there. All the people we saw there are very tall. We saw Nephilim there. (The descendants of Anak are Nephilim.) We felt as small as grasshoppers, and that's how we must have looked to them'" (Numbers 13:31-33).

Caleb and Joshua, however, had a different perspective:

> "At the same time, two of those who had explored the land, Joshua (son of Nun) and Caleb (son of Jephunneh), tore their clothes in despair. They said to the whole community of Israel, 'The land we explored is very good. If the Lord is pleased with us, He will bring us into this land and give it to us. This is a land flowing with milk and honey! Don't rebel against the Lord, and don't be afraid of the people of the land. We will devour them like bread. They have no protection, and the Lord is with us. So don't be afraid of them'" (Numbers 14:6-9).

Cancer patients, their loved ones, and caregivers are like these spies. They live close to the border and get a glimpse of the Promised Land. As we trust our Lord Jesus, we can, like Caleb and Joshua, look forward to, rather than fear, the Promised Land. Let us echo their words, "He (the Lord) will bring us into this land" … "So don't be afraid" (Numbers 14:8 & 9).

Let us not drop the mic about this message. The world fears talk about entrance to the Promised Land (death), but we don't. We look forward to an eternal Kingdom where there is no more death, fear, illness, or tears.

That's our message. Don't Drop the Mic!

87 My Life Verse

Lesson Learned, Opportunity Opened, or Purpose Pursued:

> I Have One Task Left!

Early on in this journey, I adopted a new "life verse" to guide the rest of my life. This verse is Acts 20:24:

> "I consider my life worth nothing to me, if only I may finish the race and complete the task the Lord Jesus has given me—the task of testifying to the Gospel of God's grace."

Dear Heavenly Father, please help me to recognize that my life has worth only in relationship to You, to Your remaining purposes for my life, and to the value and righteousness You imputed to me through the death and resurrection of Your Son, Jesus Christ, my Lord and Savior. Amen.

Part Three— Reflections from a Caregiver

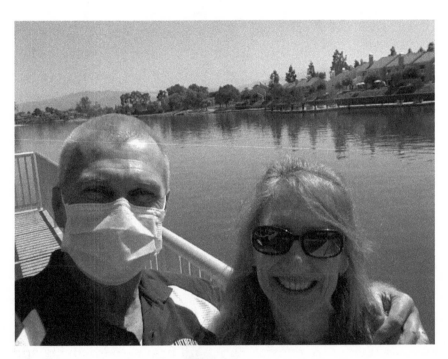

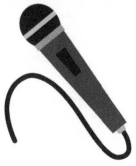

88 Joy & Peace in the Midst

Lesson Learned, Opportunity Opened, or Purpose Pursued by the Caregiver:

> "May the God of Hope Fill You with all Joy and Peace as You Trust in Him, so that You May Overflow with Hope by the Power of the Holy Spirit." Romans 15:13

Inevitably, at some point during the journey of caring for someone we love who has cancer, we will face the reality of our inadequacy to meet the myriad needs of our loved one – let alone even our own needs.

Add to the concerns and demands of caring for a loved one, long days, short nights of sleep, uncertainties about the future, multitudinous demands and responsibilities, and more, sooner or later we realize we just can't keep doing this—at least on our own.

And the last thing our loved ones need is for us to be needy, too. They need us to be full to overflowing with hope in Christ by the power of the Holy Spirit so that we can be used by the Lord to help meet their greatest need in the midst of the difficult journey – to trust in Jesus and to hold on to the hope we have in Him.

Thankfully, we have a loving, gracious God Who is more than able to meet every need our loved ones or we may face. He stands by us waiting for us to invite Him to **fill us up—with all joy and peace** as we trust in Him. As we trust Him, we will be filled to overflowing so that His joy and peace will flow into and through us to bless others, and especially to bless our loved ones for whom we are caring.

Jesus alone is the source of all joy and peace as we trust in Him!

89 It's Not About You

Lesson Learned, Opportunity Opened, or Purpose Pursued by the Caregiver:

> "This is How We Know what Love is: Jesus Christ Laid Down His life for Us. And We Ought to Lay Down our Lives for our Brothers and Sisters." 1 John 3:16

"It's not about you" is the stunning reminder with which Rick Warren begins his best-selling book, <u>The Purpose Driven Life</u>.

Caregivers (along with all followers of Christ) must come to grips with that reality, and what blessings are found in that reality! Most caregivers will usually experience the way that family, friends, and acquaintances frequently check on, pray for, and send encouragement to the one who is sick – and so they should. But few are the ones who remember also to check on, pray for, and encourage the caregiver—and that is okay.

That is okay; in fact, it is a blessing, because caregivers are called by the Lord to a very special calling—to discover in a new and deeper way what love is.

In 1 John 3:16, we are told what love is: Jesus Christ laid down His life for us. And we are privileged to lay down our lives for our brothers or sisters.

No, we don't really fully lay down our lives in caregiving, but we are privileged to come to a fuller understanding of Christ's sacrificial love and the true joy that is ours in loving with His love, in living for Him, and in recognizing the smallness of a life about me, and the fullness of a life in which it's all about Him!

90 Fear or Faith

Lesson Learned, Opportunity Opened, or Purpose Pursued by the Caregiver:

"I am The Lord, Your God, Who Takes Hold of Your Right Hand and Says to You, Do Not Fear; I Will Help You." Isaiah 41:13

When my then-thirty-three-year-old husband came home and said, "They think it's cancer," fear overwhelmed me. We had two small children, were just about to move into a brand new house, and knew a very uncertain future loomed before us.

How were we going to manage the move, the children, surgeries, treatments, hospitalizations, and myriad unknowns! Then the grace of God washed over me and the Holy Spirit gave me a peace as I realized and said to my husband, "We do know what the future holds, but we know Who holds the future."

We had a choice: focus on all the fears that were going through our minds, or focus on the Lord Who, not only holds the future but, promises to hold our hand and says to us "Do not fear; I will help you." And in ways we could never have imagined, He did help us, provide for us, and even bless us on the journey.

Fear or faith. You cannot have it both ways! Either we can choose to live in fear with anxiety about the journey or we can live by faith with peace as we trust God Who does hold our hand and helps us. Fear and faith are mutually exclusive; either you will live in fear, or you will live by faith.

That first diagnosis of my husband's cancer was over thirty years ago. By God's amazing grace, he was blessed to enjoy a thirty-year reprieve from cancer, until another devastating diagnosis of cancer. We continue to face the uncertainties that are inherent in the treatment trail, and we have the choice: live in fear or live by faith. Our many life experiences through the intervening years have taught us that we can choose to live by faith and experience the "peace that passes understanding" as we journey down the treatment trail with the Lord holding on to our hand, reminding us, "Do not fear; I will help you." The Lord is faithful, and by faith, we trust that our future is in His hands.

91 His Grace is Sufficient

Lesson Learned, Opportunity Opened, or Purpose Pursued by the Caregiver:

He Said to Me, "My Grace is Sufficient for you, for My Power is Made Perfect in Weakness." 2 Corinthians 12:9

As we faced my husband's third diagnosis of cancer with the only option for treatment, at the time, being a stem cell transplant, we began learning about the long, arduous treatment trail ahead involving:

- Three more in-patient cycles of chemotherapy
- Surgical insertion of a central venous catheter
- Moving into auxiliary housing near the hospital for at least two weeks before the stem cell transplant in the hospital and an undetermined length after the transplant
- Stem cell collection every day for nine days
- Hospitalization for almost three weeks for high-dose chemotherapy to eradicate his immune system
- Infusion of his stem cells
- And the long recovery of his immune system, and so much more!

Caregiving, at this point, moved to a whole new level for me, including:

- Moving up to the auxiliary housing to care for him
- Providing meals for him in our hotel room due to his being in isolation
- Being essentially in isolation myself to protect him
- Sitting by his side through infusions of "toxic" chemotherapy drugs (The nurses wore gloves, gowns, and masks, while I had none of those protections! After sitting next to Bill for literally dozens of chemotherapy treatments,

I even began to experience slight side-effects—imaginary, empathetic, or real—of the drugs!)
- Traveling three-plus hours each day during the hospitalization times to sit with him
- Learning to give him twice-daily injections
- Cleaning every square inch of the house with disinfectants before his homecoming, and on and on.

I write this, not to complain but, to acknowledge the untold challenges facing those who provide the care and support for those they love—recognizing that caregiving has its own challenges in the treatment trail. Some days, caregivers are stretched almost to the breaking point, emotionally (with concerns for our loved ones) and physically (with all the needs the caregivers strive to meet).

How does a caregiver not only cope but find strength and even blessings for the journey?

We turn to the Lord and His promises, such as 2 Corinthians 12:9 in which He reminds us that His grace is sufficient and His power is made perfect in weakness. In our weakness, we are forced to rely on Christ and His power, and we discover that His grace truly is sufficient.

Each morning we begin the day by reading God's Word and praying, and during the cancer treatment trail, we began a wonderful habit of writing down three blessings from the day before—three reminders of how His grace truly was (and will be) sufficient for each day.

We began to realize how the Lord abundantly and faithfully met our needs every step of the way. A few of the many amazing examples include:
- His provision of a generous offer from a neighborhood gardener (who had just cut trees in our yard before) to mow our yard at no charge for us for the months my husband was unable to do this

- Our Lord's provision of my sister's availability to help with my mother during the time I needed to stay with my husband to care for him at the auxiliary housing by the hospital after the transplant. My sister, who lives out of town, had a week off of work that enabled her to be with my 93-year-old mother with dementia at the hospital after her fall and surgery when I couldn't be there.
- New and effective treatments options surfaced within weeks of our being told that we had no additional options after the stem cell treatment (which did not "take"), and so many more examples of His faithful provision that we could fill a book!

The Lord has shown us daily that His grace is sufficient and His power is made perfect in our weakness. He will supply the strength, the courage, the help, or whatever our need may be. He is faithful, and we can trust Him.

> "That is why, for Christ's sake, I delight in weaknesses, in insults, in hardships, in persecutions, in difficulties. For when I am weak, then I am strong" (2 Corinthians 12:10).

92 You Are More Than a Bone Marrow Biopsy!

Lesson Learned, Opportunity Opened, or Purpose Pursued by the Caregiver:

> "See What Great Love the Father has Lavished on Us, that We Should be Called Children of God! And That is What We Are!" 1 John 3:1

One of the most encouraging conversations I had with my caregiver (my wife, Cindy!) occurred after a bone marrow biopsy that I dreaded, endured, and survived at the beginning of the clinical trial. I still vividly remember lying on my stomach, lower back exposed, doctor readying the long and infamous bone marrow biopsy needle, and then asking me, "What do you do, Mr. Bartlett?"

My present circumstance dictated a duplicitous response. Outwardly, and in a calm voice, I replied to the doctor, "Oh, not much other than treatment these days." Inwardly, I was screaming, "What do you think I am doing! I am lying flat on a table about to have a needle jammed into my backside and pushed into my bone! That's what I'm doing!"

The doctor, of course, heard my outward (and polite) response and replied, "You are more than just a patient. What else do you do?"

What an insightful statement. There was a silent pause among us all—the doctor, my wife, and me. Then, I shared a little of what I had done as a pastor and educator, but still missed the point of her question as she was inquiring as to what I was doing now. The searing indictment was more painful than the biopsy needle.

I did survive that bone marrow biopsy—and it was not bad at all, so please forget any of those stories about how bad such a procedure is! On the way home that day, Cindy and I had a conversation about the doctor's question, my answer, and the doctor's reply to my answer.

In our culture, the question "What do you do?" is often an accepted form of asking, "Who are you?"

My response to the doctor of saying, "Oh, not much more than treatment these days," prompted a comment from my wife. Cindy said, "The doctor was right. You are more than just a patient."

I agreed. I also confessed the "inner voice" that screamed, "What do you think I am doing...."

Between the disarming response of the doctor, my wife's comment, and my own confession, a lesson was taught that day—a lesson that I frequently remember, and a lesson that regularly still causes me to pause and thank the Lord for the doctor's reminder and, even more so, to thank the Lord for the gift of being His child.

The next time I am asked, "What do you do?"—whether I'm flat on my stomach waiting for a bone marrow biopsy (again, remember, it really wasn't that bad!) or simply in a casual conversation, I now have a ready response:

- I'm a child of God!
- I share His love and joy!
- I reflect His peace!
- I pray for His Will!
- I love others with the love He has first given me!
- I am a servant of Jesus!
- I am a student, daily learning lessons about life and eternity!
- I respond with His grace to opportunities daily opened!
- I am a person with passion and purpose for Christ!
- I am a laborer for God's coming Kingdom!
- I have a very full life!

I love what I do! It is a gift and a privilege from our Lord!

Now, let me ask you, "What do you do?" Specifically, what will you do with the lessons learned, the opportunities opened, and purposes to pursue revealed on this treatment trail?

May we together, in words and deeds, echo the life-mission that Apostle Paul articulated in Acts 20:24:

> "I consider my life worth nothing to me; my only aim is to finish the race and complete the task the Lord Jesus has given me—the task of testifying to the Good News of God's grace."

Part Four—Epilogue: QR Codes for Joining the Dialog

Use a QR reader app (on your phone) for the following images. Once you have the web addresses on your phone, you can email them to your computer or tablet to bookmark for ease of access.

Access Pastor Bartlett's ongoing "Lessons Learned, Opportunities Opened, and Purposes Pursued on the Treatment Trail," including links to referenced supporting info and documents.

Lessons, Opportunities, and Purpose continue!

Join the discussion in a "Cancer: Don't Drop the Mic" Forum/Blog to make a post, to reply to others, or to share your thoughts.

https://dontdropthemic.wordpress.com/

Don't Drop the Mic! Keep the Dialogue Alive!

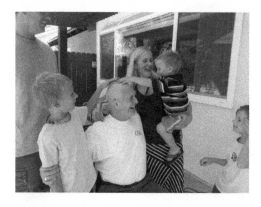